"Moving, inspiring, and poetically written, *Back to Life* belongs in the hands of anyone who has gone through a difficult patch in life, or cares about someone who has. We all hope to transit the major challenges of life with honesty and grace. This book is a model of how to do just that."

— Lance M. Dodes, M.D., Assistant Clinical Professor of Psychiatry, Harvard Medical School Training and Supervising Analyst, Boston Psychoanalytic Society and Institute

"Medical trauma is an overwhelming and terrifying experience. Pamela Douglas' book on the trauma of back surgery both informs and tells a story — all the while holding the reader's hand. For what is inspiration if not the ability to comfort during a time of fear? Ms. Douglas has found the language that tenderly and bravely describes the human journey through medical trauma, resulting in a document that maps the way through tragedy and loss to triumph and celebration."

— Alesia Willow Montana, MA, LPC, CSAC, Trauma Therapist

"In today's world, patients long for instant cures. They are often dismayed that healing after spine surgery takes time. This is especially true for patients undergoing corrective surgery for scoliosis. Douglas has drawn on her personal experience with scoliosis surgery. She thoughtfully and successfully provides a guidebook for patients contemplating this procedure by verbalizing doubts and fears and offering a realistic framework of appropriate expectations, both positive and negative. Her personal and sensitive approach in communicating these expectations successfully enables individuals contemplating such surgery to make a more informed decision."

— Steven M. Wetzner, M.D., Emeritus Chairman of Radiology, New England Baptist Hospital Clinical Professor of Radiology, Tufts University School of Medicine

"In *Back to Life*, Pamela Douglas realistically portrays the simultaneous feelings of worry and hope that emerge in finding out one requires surgery of this magnitude. In writing her story in the format of a journal, she allows the reader to feel as if they are walking the path of transformation with her, following her thought patterns, and taking the necessary steps in preparing for a daunting, life-changing event. Additionally, Douglas provides real and useful suggestions for individuals who may have back surgery in the future and illustrates how it is possible to realize incredible strength one might never have known they had."

— Shawna Delaney, Lead Social Skills Instructor, Autism Spectrum Therapies

"Pamela Douglas chose to have a very difficult back surgery and, having chosen it, she tells the story with clarity, wry humor, and an eye for the practical. Behind this, though she doesn't point it out, stands her courage. That and the love of a very dear family can inspire the rest of us who also have mortal challenges. Here's how to face them."

    — Beverly Pierce, MLS, MA, RN, CHTP, The Institute for Integrative
      Health

"A light read about a difficult endeavor, both physically and psychologically. A real down-to-earth anecdotal account of going through back surgery and how to cope with it all. Ms. Douglas provides us with a positive model for enduring the ups and downs."

    — Dr. Susan F. Rabin, Ph.D., CCCJS, DAC, CDVC, MFT

"An unflinchingly honest portrait of facing life's biggest and toughest questions."

    — Donna Freitas, Ph.D., columnist and blogger for BeliefNet.com,
      author of several books, including *Sex and the Soul: Juggling Sexuality,*
      Spirituality, Romance, and Religion on America's College Campuses, pub-
      lished by Oxford University Press

"A vital resource for anyone contemplating Adult Scoliosis surgery."

    — Terrence T. Kim, M.D., Orthopaedic Spine Surgeon, Cedars-Sinai
      Spine Center, Los Angeles, CA

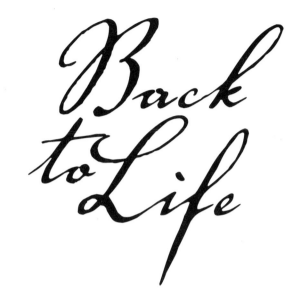

Back to Life

A

JOURNEY OF

TRANSFORMATION

THROUGH BACK

SURGERY

Pamela Douglas

DIVINE
ARTS

Published by DIVINE ARTS
DivineArtsMedia.com

An imprint of Michael Wiese Productions
12400 Ventura Blvd. #1111
Studio City, CA 91604
(818) 379-8799, (818) 986-3408 (FAX)

Cover design by Johnny Ink. www.johnnyink.com
Copyediting by Marsha D. Phillips
Book Layout by William Morosi
Printed by McNaughton & Gunn, Inc., Saline, Michigan

Manufactured in the United States of America

Library of Congress Cataloging-in-Publication Data

Douglas, Pamela
  Back to life : a journey of transformation through back surgery / Pamela Douglas.
     p. cm.
  Summary: "Close-up and personal, this book brings readers into the day-to-day, even minute-
by-minute, experience of preparing for, undergoing, and recovering from life-threatening spine
surgery. Written in the form of a journal, the brief entries offer both the immediacy of a realistic
drama and a transcendent peek into the transformational power that this surgery represented
for the writer"-- Provided by publisher.
  ISBN 978-1-61125-002-2 (pbk.)
  1. Douglas, Pamela --- Health. 2. Spine--Diseases--Patients--California--Biography. 3. Spine--
Surgery. I. Title.
  RD768.D68 2011
  617.5'6059092--dc22
  [B]
                                    2011002828

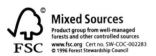

Mixed Sources
Product group from well-managed
forests and other controlled sources
www.fsc.org Cert no. SW-COC-002283
© 1996 Forest Stewardship Council

Hexagram 32
HÊNG : THE LONG ENDURING

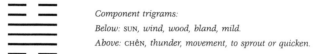

Component trigrams:
Below: SUN, *wind, wood, bland, mild.*
Above: CHÊN, *thunder, movement, to sprout or quicken.*

"...Every end is succeeded by a new beginning.... The four seasons, with their ceaseless transformations, are able to produce their effects for eons. The inner nature of everything in heaven and earth can be judged from contemplating whatever it is that makes them continue to be as they are."

> — John Blofeld, trans., commentary to
> *I Ching: The Book of Change (circa 1150 BC)*

Table of Contents

≈

Preface

≈

FOR THE FIRST TIME, I had to make a life-threatening medical decision. My spine was collapsing. It had curved out from a 49-degree bend just five years ago, to a bulge of 70 degrees. If I did nothing, the degeneration would likely increase until my spine pressed on my internal organs, my breathing would be compromised, and I would live the rest of my life in a wheelchair.

The choice to fix my spine seemed simple. But this was anything but simple. There would be two surgeries: one cutting into my front to saw off a rib — to remove many of my spinal discs and fuse the vertebrae — on the first long day. The second operation, two days later, would be to cut all the way down my back, placing large metal screws in my vertebrae to hold steel rods that would prop up my spine. Then I'd be walled into a heavy body brace for months afterwards and wouldn't be completely healed for a year. That's, of course, if it worked. That's if (as my doctors were careful to inform me) I didn't have serious complications — including death.

Statistically, death, paralysis and other disasters, combined, are around one percent. That may not seem too bad, but it's a whole lot worse than sitting in a wheelchair.

Still, even if I survived, the prospects were frightening. When I told a friend I was considering this surgery, her hand flew to her mouth and she pleaded with me not to do it. She'd known someone who'd suffered terribly after back surgery with pain that disabled her completely. "Horrific" was her word.

So which way to go?

I had to focus on decisions many of us avoid: Who would "pull the plug" in the worst case? This is a question I was forced to answer because the hospital required an Advanced Directive. I found myself brooding over how to provide for my daughter in my absence. But I also had to imagine the burden on my husband and daughter if I let my condition degenerate to the point that I was unable to walk or work, or I was drugged-out on pain-killers, or if I postponed the surgery until it was too far gone to correct.

Though I wasn't aware of it at the time, on an ephemeral level, I was ready for the next step — a transformation, whatever that might be — even urgent for it. On a pragmatic level, confidence in my surgeon and the support of my family led to the operation.

The surgery wasn't smooth — I lost so much blood I required two transfusions. My heart had to be stabilized, landing me in Intensive Care for four days after my second operation. One of my lungs collapsed in the first surgery, and I couldn't get out of bed by myself or walk for weeks.

But I made it through. Finally, I even did well. I was changed in ways both small and profound. And I want to share my journey with anyone it may help.

Introduction

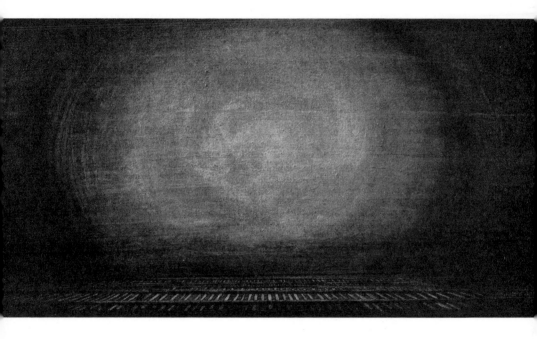

I DESPERATELY WANTED TO KNOW.

In a few months I was headed for spine surgery and I couldn't put it off any longer. Now I *had* to know. Not the medical facts — I could find those on my surgeon's website, on the internet, and in technical books by doctors. No, I needed the personal feel of what I'd be going through, how to get ready, what I'd experience in the hospital, and the day by day struggle to reclaim a normal life, if "normal" would ever mean what it had before. Who could tell me?

I asked everyone: my doctor; my exercise teacher; relatives who vaguely knew someone who had back surgery; and all my acquaintances. But, when I contacted people who'd had the surgery, as generous as they were, I couldn't invade the privacy of strangers. Nor did they want to remember.

That's why I wrote this book. As I went through the process I kept notes as close to my experiences as possible. If I'd waited even a few weeks, the details would have drifted like dandelion seeds in the wind.

A World of Back Trouble

As bipeds, we humans tend to have aching backs, but rather than return to walking on all fours, we devise other solutions for the pain. Bookstores overflow with therapies like massage, yoga, and meditation. One store owner told me that self-help for back pain is second only to tips for weight loss. But serious structural problems like scoliosis (an excessive curvature of the spine, which is what I have), and degenerating discs, can't be fixed by massage or positive thinking — believe me, I've tried.

When it's that bad, doctors have to operate, and half a million back surgeries are performed each year, including thousands of spine fusions like mine. A little extra bend in the back is common and usually doesn't lead to surgery. But an extreme S-curve, or curves that press on internal organs, or that make a side, chest, or back bulge out, land people on operating tables.

No one knows what causes scoliosis — maybe some genetic predisposition or an imbalance during growth. And no one has a cure, only ways of stabilizing the spine. The surgeon fuses the vertebrae as straight as possible and places steel rods beside the spine, held with metal screws, into the bones. That's what happened to me.

My Own Journey

I first learned the word *scoliosis* when I was diagnosed in college, but I did just fine for decades, having a baby, a career, a garden, and actually using my gym membership. But as time went on so did my curve, finally leaning so much that my ribs were bumping into my pelvis when I bent and a kind of hump was visible. Still, I didn't want to think about it.

Take six months out of my schedule for surgery? You gotta be kidding! I was too busy. I'm on the faculty of the School of Cinematic Arts at the University of Southern California (USC), where I teach screenwriting, and I'm a working writer. In fact, my book, *Writing the TV Drama Series*, had just been accepted for publication when I first met with the surgeon. I needed to be available to proofread the galleys and promote the book. I'd also recently returned to painting. And I take care of a household. No way, no way, nooo waaaay was I going to stop my life to do — what? Get all cut up and turn into a cyborg with steel parts? Nooooo.

I considered the perspective that we are all "transhumans," a term invented by futurist F.M. Esfandiary (FM 2030). He meant anyone who has dental work, or wears glasses or hearing aids — not to mention all those with heart stents or hip or knee replacements — are part non-biological. That stretches the idea of what it means to be human. What part of us remains? But surely the very vortex of vital life force, the cosmic energy moving through the nerve ganglia attached to the spine — that should be untouched. Aren't the paths of those impulses too close to the definition of who we are?

I thought hard about this choice, knowing that change is the only constant in life. The unknown — and change always produces unknowns — threatens our fantasy that we are in control of our lives.

So if you imagine, as I do, that on an unseen level all things are connected, then any change, however slight, changes everything. A dramatic change to my body would have ramifications beyond what all the gauges and monitors and labs in a hospital can measure. The greater question, then, was not how my body would adjust, but how my world might be different.

That's daunting. I told myself that I take calculated risks every time I cross the street, drive a car, or step in a bathtub. Still, I go on and do what I must. But really, I just wasn't sure.

Then one day while I was getting a haircut, a cautionary tale played out before me. A sophisticated, vigorous woman I'd noticed in the salon for years hobbled into the room grotesquely bent, barely able to walk, on the arm of a caregiver. She was around seventy, though I hadn't thought about her age because she had always been so active.

She explained that one morning she'd tried to get out of bed and suddenly her lower body was paralyzed. Alone and unable to reach a phone, she sat for hours until a neighbor heard her screaming. Without warning, her spine had collapsed overnight. Well, it wasn't completely without warning. She'd been told her discs were gradually degenerating, but she didn't consider that an emergency, and she was planning a cruise. Now it was too late. Her condition was too far gone, her heart too weak, so surgery was impossible. Someone would have to help her twenty-four hours a day for the rest of her life.

That did it. What was losing a few months from my job and my creative work compared to a lifetime spent incapacitated? Thus, I met with Dr. Robert Pashman, M.D., Director of the Scoliosis and Spinal Deformity Institute at Cedars-Sinai Medical Center in Los Angeles. Though it was early fall 2004, I went ahead and scheduled surgery for mid-May 2005, more than six months in advance, to coincide with the end of teaching for the year. I needed time to resolve practical issues like arranging a disability leave and making sure my health insurance would cover everything. And I didn't feel it would be right to ditch my students in the middle of the term.

I prepared my family, decided which work to finish and what didn't matter, and most of all, I consciously found joy in familiar patterns that were about to change.

About this Book

I asked myself what kind of book I'd want to read to guide me through, and remembered the baby books I'd consumed while I was pregnant and after my daughter was born. Back then, I'd hungered to know if each twinge and pang was normal. Even more fascinating were the toddler charts — at this month they smile, then they say mama, crawled at this time, the first step by that month. Moms all over hang on those milestones for signs their progeny is precocious or to know when to freak and call the pediatrician. I used to dwell on the case studies showing how other babies ate or moved or what worked to stop them from crying.

With that model, I began writing this book two months before my surgery and continued until four months after I was out of the hospital. So here is half a year of pain and joy, humor and rage, discoveries, reflections, and fitful increments of hard won progress.

I've also included the voices of my family because they lived this experience almost as much as I did. My daughter, Raya Yarbrough, kept a journal which I didn't see until months after I was out of the hospital — a moving, literary expression in its own right.

Step-by-step details of each operation, as explained by my surgeon's technician, appear in the hospital section. The process he and the doctor described left me in awe, not only of the procedure, but of the body's ability to heal after such a thing.

I'm not a doctor or a nurse. I make no claim to medical expertise, and I'm not prescribing medical remedies. Dr. Pashman suggested an additional disclaimer: I'm not typical because I was in better general health than many people who come to him, so my recovery was quicker and easier than what some other patients might experience.

But this book is not only about a serious operation; it also offers insights into how one family coped, and it's about transformation. For anyone going through a medical challenge, this book may speak to you.

For me, the result was worth the hardships. At the end I feel stronger than when I began. I wish that for you too.

Before

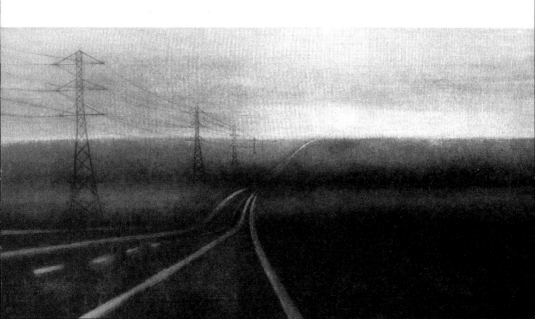

≈

Chasing Joy

Every precious step, I love every errand with the wholeness of a person intact, able to go, do. The familiar is about to become alien so I chase the happiness of a simple walk — the step, step, step itself — not "taking a walk" in any romantic sense of enjoying a park. No, what I am clinging to is the feel of the sidewalk, the miracle of judging traffic to know if you can get across before a car skims the ground going places. Going places. Everyone going. Yes, to the supermarket. Yes, through the parking lot. Yes, to the aisle with the coffee. Yes, the colors in the aisle, the smells. The sheer power, the freedom to go on those simple errands — every day I love it all.

The Family Visit

"Have you seen her X-ray?" the doctor asked my daughter Raya and my husband John Spencer, and trooped us off to behold the sideshow of my bulging, twisted spine naked in white light on the black screen in a small dark room. He moved the computer pointer, drawing white lines across the vertebrae marked with numbers of ignominy: 70 degrees, 49 degrees, numbers that said it will not continue to hold me up.

"I'd feel better about this if you were in pain. Most of the people who come in here are in terrible pain," the doctor said.

But I'm fine. I looked at him, upright, the kind of guy who got all A's in school and trounced all opposition without a flinch. Tall, good-looking, no doubt rich, smart. John said later, that's the best thing going for me, this doctor's ego that he has to be perfect, the best, that he has to win, and I'm his raw material to make right.

Raya wanted to know the details — what would be done, every cut, every change. He didn't really have time. Look at the website.

"Do you really want to know?" he asked, surprised. He'd send in his tech if we did.

That's all right, we said.

So we came home, the three of us in his hands, having been told it would all work out, though we'd been given the printed disclosure form listing the terrible risks. We went home with nothing more to say, feeling like three small people with only each other. It's not as if we could complain: we'd been given specific answers to the questions we could put into words. As if it were easy.

March 19

≈

Martha Stewart

She spent five months in jail — the same amount of time I will be unable to drive, and will be confined, like her, to a limited space; like her, absent from the things that had defined her. In Martha's case, she couldn't be home for holidays, but she moved about the grounds picking crabapples, I read.

Why be obsessed with her as she enters prison just months before I go into the hospital? Surely, we have so little in common — her empire, her life waiting, barely changed, or even improved after it's over. I'm told I'll be changed forever. When I'm out of "house arrest" I'll never be free from the internal cage around my spine. That's what they call it, a cage, necessary for me to walk straight, "straighten up and fly right." My incarceration will be internal, and the question I can't know until it's over is: what freedom will I have later?

Plans

Details of the future. You make plans that seem to take account of the vicissitudes. You create ways of coping. A certain day and hour is the blood bank donation, or the appointment with the internist, or the vascular specialist. You make plans to get a walker and an extra rubber bathmat or two so the shower won't be slippery. Plans for disability pay so the world will keep turning — the house, the car, so Raya and John will have groceries. I'm planning to make a schedule for when I'm not here: when to water the plants, to wash the sheets.

But the schedule can go only so far. Don't need to water the plants until I'm home, but in the event ... water once a month. In the event.... The life insurance number is ... and would the pension pay anything? And how long would any of that last?

Providers

Since cave days, women have provided (different from men who went out to shoot beasts or bring things home) the objects of a home. It was the women who provided sustenance, the content of the home, the heart, the reason for staying together. Sometimes it seems we are still in that cave. So what if a woman cannot provide?

I spend these weeks before entering the hospital devising ways to care-take in my absence. Not just how to work the dishwasher, not just the groceries and my idea of over-filling the fridge the weekend before I leave — I plan for all the unknown days that might follow because, the truth is, I don't know.

"What if" looms over me, a vise that I deny, but I know that if I am to provide, I need to look at everything and say: *Now*. Now I will do everything while I can. So I call the pension, and the life insurance, and the benefits department at work, and every other sanctuary set up to cover a time when someone else may need to provide. I hope they can, but I know that in my absence, no matter how well they supply the things of a household — money, artifacts — they'd be left with a hollow shell of our home.

Puzzle Pieces

The doctor explained he was going to take out the discs and set them aside, push away my intestines and other organs, leaving me a shell where metal rods would hold up the remaining carcass. "I", the mind that once was embodied, would be retrofitted and set back in motion, re-booted, or maybe it would be like turning the water and power back on after a siege.

So who am I in all this? An unconscious bystander (sorry, bysleeper), the inhabitant of someone who was, whose form had changed? I'd be set down in an altered body and told I am continuous, that nothing happened except that the pieces of the puzzle had been removed and put back — well, most put back, some new, but that the puzzle still matched the picture on the box.

Still, as I wrote my name on this journal, as I will write my name on the hospital admissions, as I will sign permission for all this to occur, I hold dear to the person who was linked to the child, the adolescent, the young mother, the person at a first job, to my parents who made the original. And then I'll prepare for who I will become.

April 10

≈

Rage

For two weeks I've been raging: anger at the long line in the post office (thirty people in line and one clerk who puts up a closed sign); anger at the car in front of me on the freeway, poking along at 50 mph in the fast lane; most of all, rage at the disability office for being confused, obstinate, slow to process my claim for benefits when I start my medical leave just five weeks from now.

Twenty-three years working for this place, paying into their disability program, twenty-three years of deductions from my paychecks, 23 x 12 paychecks and still they resist giving me any disability pay over the summer and agree only to "consider" after they see medical records later. Rage. Rage that they responded to the doctor's letter asking for my leave until the winter term by defining winter as starting on August 15th. The office urged me to calm down, that it would all be taken care of. Maybe so.

But the rage continues: anger that I feel powerless, at the ultimate loss of power when I'm lying unconscious under utter control of men with knives, fury that I cannot defend myself against this invasion, and that no one, nothing, can quell my days of fury.

Doubts

A lawyer friend described surgeons as arrogant. "They make a good living for themselves, especially if they do lots of these. Have you had a second opinion?"

Yes, of course. The rival doctor said my spine was degenerating and I need to have this operation sooner or later, better sooner, when I can get well.

But the Pilates teacher also dangled doubt: "You're getting more flexible; maybe you don't have to...."

What good does all that do unless I would actually turn around, stop the wheels in motion now. I could. People leave grooms at the altar. People flee for their lives on the eve of a disaster. And people persevere and do follow a decision, and ultimately they're better for it — or not.

On this day when I bought a walker to help me stand in the shower; on this day when I got the Advanced Directive notarized, saying that if I died they could transplant my body parts but not my eyes (sorry, not my eyes); on this day when I arranged for the paralegal to do my will, just in case.... On this day of preparing, I don't want the doubts that whisper at me to turn back from the precipice: "You don't have to do this." Or do I?

Asking

I've been asking everyone for reassurance. Do you know any-body who's had it done? Their stories always tell me what I already know.

"I knew a woman," the receptionist at Pilates said, "she was all bent over so she was walking around facing the floor. The doctors said it was affecting her internal organs so she *had* to get the operation. She was 55 when she did it. Why did she wait so long?" the receptionist wondered.

I pressed her, "How did she do?"

"Terrible at first," she answered. "The woman was so sick and that went on for two months. The pain. But it wasn't only the pain. She was sick, you know, she felt sick all the time."

I pressed further, "But after two months she was all right?"

She took Pilates, the receptionist explained and after a lot of rehab she did better, as long as she kept it up for the rest of her life.

"But she was all right after the Pilates?" I was pushing her.

"Yes, she was all right after a while."

So when it was all behind her, she was better, she was fine, I insisted.

The receptionist looked at me kindly, "Yes, after awhile it was all over and she was fine."

April 13

〜

Unfinished Work

I'm reluctant to start a new painting — keep postponing buying the paints and even touching the surface with a preliminary sketch, for fear I won't be able to finish in time. Barely more than a month, but a subtle painting can take a month or more. What if the work is awkward two days before I leave? Or what if I leave it unfinished? Without what I meant to say? Dare I start? I sound like T.S. Eliot's poem: "The Lovesong of J. Alfred Prufrock" ("Should I presume?"). But it's tangible now.

Today I finally planted a seedling I've been nurturing into my potted plant in my office at school. It was a big effort, lugging the heavy bag of soil from the parking lot, cutting it open with the receptionist's scissors, and scooping the soil into the pot, its earthy scent infusing the office where my esteemed colleague was trying to read. I took that seedling and settled its roots on new soft soil, filled the pot, and put it back on top of the book-case. It was important, urgent, to do it now or the seedling won't have settled before I bring the plants home. I'll have to bring them home because I won't be around to take care. Who would water them when I'm gone? I couldn't let that go unfinished, just as I hesitate to begin anything new.

Before my mother died she said, "Thank you," though I didn't really understand why until now. She wanted nothing left unfinished, and that was good.

April 22

≈

From Raya's Journal

She is not the one leaving. I am. After mama's operation, this is the last big care I will give her in my young life. This is the last part of my childhood shoving off. This is the daughter preparing to be the mother to her mother, and then — to leave. I will be moving out in the next year or so, but also moving on.

I had a vision in the waking hours this morning. I saw my mother in bed at home after the operation. She looked skinny but not terribly, and it was a relief to see a moment of "after." The expression on her face was a quiet shock, an attempt to rationalize and hold together a completely alien situation — the kind of shock that moves in slow motion over a long time — the sound of glass breaking as if it were liquefied, stretched out and lapping at your ears in serrated waves.

April 23

≈

Trees

Lately I've wanted to paint a tree, looking up with wonder at the branches that would embrace me, set in the midst of arms greater than mine, affirming the long lifetime it takes to grow a tree that is grand. It's easy to draw trees, and though all my paintings begin with non-representational colors, rhythms and structure, I've found living, growing forms in them before — a single tall lily, a tree whose roots reach deep into the shape of the earth.

This was a simple impulse, so why was it so difficult? The tree I created had no balance, and it was odd, reaching rigidly but never finding its life. Why was I having trouble with this one painting, a work that wouldn't have been special, a square wooden panel with textures? Why was I suddenly unable to create this most basic element? Finally, shapes of birds rose up one side and the trunk was inhabited by the suggestion of a figure, lying, as I might lie on an operating table, naked and sprawled, embedded in the larger image. Still, the painting doesn't work.

It's time to move on. Next painting. Next step: letting go of old clothes and easy solutions. It's getting closer to the time to let go.

April 29

~

Quiet

Oddly quiet in the house though I can hear the dishwasher distant in the kitchen, a good sound of life continuing. John is asleep and Raya is out with her boyfriend. It's not unusual, really, but everything seems hushed now all day, the unspoken, as we go about our routines.

Today I packed copies of my will in three white envelopes. I gave one to Raya and told her to put it at the bottom of a drawer and not even bother looking at it, and watched as she closed the drawer on it, folded in half, shut. I'll mail one to Cathy, my "exec-utress," my friend. After all the years and people I've known, it turned out she was the one I trusted, though we rarely see each other and our original connection was more than twenty years ago when our children were babies together in a mommy-and-me group, at a time I didn't imagine I would ever stop being a mommy holding hands in a circle with tiny children.

Today it's quiet, no small children, no one here, a sense of inevitability, acceptance. My teaching term is over, no more students, no more papers to read, no meetings, no issues to debate or faculty diatribes at someone who wanted a different syllabus or schedule than someone else wanted. Think of that: someone who wanted something. Not a lot to want in the quiet, except the simple routines we use to keep life going to fill the quiet.

April 30

≈

Wheelchair

Almost twenty years ago a chiropractor told me that one day I'd be in a wheelchair: "progressive, incurable degeneration of the spine." It was only a matter of time, he said, though I was a young mother then, too busy starting my career and raising a child to do anything about it. But I've carried the ominous prediction with me all these years, glad for every step I've taken. For me, walking to mail a letter at the corner is a celebration, and not a single day do I get out of bed, on my own feet, and take it for granted.

Maybe that's why I have so little pain, though people make that squished pitying face — "Does it hurt a lot?" No, it doesn't hurt at all, I tell them, and usually it doesn't because being able to walk is so much larger. And now it seems something can be done. I'll never be in a wheelchair after all (except coming out of the hospital). All the dread I've amassed staring at wheelchairs can dissipate now, if I can let it. I can't be healed, but I can be held up to walk on my own legs and never be bound by a fate that I once believed was sealed, if I had let it be.

May 1

≈

The Mink Coat

I don't wear fur — it feels like stealing someone else's skin — so I never wore my mother's mink coat. Hypocritical, I guess, because I do wear leather shoes. Still, someone's fur covering my arms gives me the creeps.

My mother never felt that way, proud of the blond mink with the shawl collar from Macy's that my father gave her — one of many gifts — usually to ask forgiveness after he'd been in a bad mood. I suppose she thought she was elegant in it, though I don't recall her wearing it.

For more than ten years since she died, that coat has hung in my closet covered in a white piece of cloth. I'd thought of selling it before and discovered that no one in Los Angeles buys what they call "vintage" fur, which is another way of saying an old coat.

But today I sold it on an ebay auction for $212.50. I found out by email in the morning when I was thinking of other things. I didn't expect to care; after all, it's not as if I'd worn it or remembered her in it especially. But now, as I'm harvesting everything I can find to cover the bills while I can't work, she has given me a present: $212.50. So I let go of her coat, though I stared at the photo on my screen too long.

Silently, I said thank you, and I felt I heard her answer, "I wish I could have given you more."

May 4 — Twelve days until....

≈

From Raya's Journal

Today we went to the blood bank for my mother to make her second donation to her cause. The operation is in about two weeks, and I should've been keeping a journal about my "deep feelings," "angst," and "profound transitional moments" for all this time, but more important things kept coming up, like a special on wall paint-sponging techniques on Channel 74.

About five minutes ago, she walked back into the "blood taking room," and I reminded her not to give all of it. I told her to mention to the nurse that she would like to keep some because we're going to lunch after this and it is my understanding that blood is necessary to the food digestion process. I impressed on her my opinion that we would look like real losers walking into Swingers without enough blood to properly deal with her meal. Aside from that, we may not have the same blood type, so I couldn't necessarily share any of my blood with her at the restaurant.

It also occurred to me that it was a waste of time for the hospital to take weeks testing my mother's blood type. I could've told them she was Type A. (I mean, just talk to her.)

May 4

≈

Blood

The TV is playing "Ambush Makeover" while the nurse inserts the needle that will run the blood out of the vein in my right arm. Banking your own blood is the safest, they say. This is my second visit to the vampire room to give a pint each time, an "autologous donor."

The first time my nurse was Leroy Brown, and today it's Mary Wilson. I think about the absurdity of pop songs from decades ago while my blood runs: "Bad, bad, Leroy Brown, baddest man in the whole damn town." And wasn't Mary Wilson one of the Supremes?

Now the "Ambush Makeover" has grabbed up an ordinary woman in jeans and brown hair and put her in a dress and high heels and cut her hair. Her friends applaud wildly and gasp at the miracle.

Yes, miracle: that they can take so much blood with so little sensation and that a plastic cup of juice will somehow replenish what I lost.

Meanwhile, Raya waits in the reception area, writing on her laptop about what's happening to me. And after, we eat at a nearby Swingers diner, and shop at a discount cowboy store across the street, though we never wear cowboy styles. Three used shirts for twenty dollars, and we're happy as she drives me home, safe now, away from the ambush. Home. Blood.

≈

From Raya's Journal

I feel like some sort of absurdist mercenary, cutting out my eyes so my head can see. I look around me and there are pamphlets with vertebrae bits colorfully rendered, bullet points to clarify surgical procedures, a stationary walker that we bought for use in the shower. But I see none of it. My eyes have been replaced with frosted glass globes into which my head is projecting rosy aurora borealis.

There is no surgery. It will be forever impending. It is just another drama my mother cooked up to worry about, but it will never happen. She will never run out of gas on the freeway, never see me married to a drug dealer, never leave the stove on and burn down the house, never get fired, and never, ever, be rendered immobile for three months with two steel rods fused to the sides of her spine.

This will not happen. My head will not allow it, and I cannot see it. It is a sci-fi fantasy of a partially bionic mother, one step better than nature's original plan. When I wake up I'll laugh at my imagination.

May 10

≈

Distractions

I've come to know too much about skirt length — that petites shouldn't wear the new full lengths because they drown you. The doctors' waiting rooms — the internist who did the pre-op labs to say I was well enough to "go under," the vascular specialist I'll see today who I'm told "will make the first cut" — all of them are framed by fashion magazines. And of course, the salon where I got my hair done this weekend, and next weekend when I have a manicure and spa pedicure, like I'm preparing for a prom.

It's not foolish vanity. This is about identity, looking in the face of becoming a patient and defiantly demonstrating "I am." I am the woman I was a year ago, a day ago, the moment before I enter that room less than a week from now. It's hard to believe as I make my grocery list to stock up on what I won't be able to go and take off the shelves myself, putting my choices, even the trivial ones, in other people's hands.

"What are you worried about?" Raya asks, as if I had a deep answer.

I tell her I worry whether the disability payment will be on time and if the rent will be mailed while I'm away.

"So you're worried whether you can count on us?"

Of course, of course I trust her and John, as I explain the bills she'll have to watch for. But she doubts the bills are truly what's bothering me. Wisely, she asks if they're just a distraction.

May 10

≈

From Raya's Journal

Sometime last year I had a dream that my father, my step-father and I were all assembled on this winding mountain pass overlooking end-less hills swathed in haze. It looked like the high passes in Malibu that eventually lead back to the sea. My mother was on a gurney on the edge of the road, a sheer cliff, and she was wrapped in white cloth except for her face. She had on her make-up; she was very comfortable, very calm.

One by one, my fathers and I were going to her side, hugging her, kissing her, and saying goodbye. The premise was that this was some sort of ultra-luxurious way to check out, that she had thought about it for a while, had looked into all of the organizations that offered this service, and that she had decided this one was the best. The back story in my head, in that timeless dream understanding, was that we had all agreed that if this was what she wanted we would let her go through with it. We had talked it over for a year and she had convinced us this was what she wanted to do.

I walked up to her, talked with her, told her goodbye. She assured me that the best thing I could do for her was to let her go. I had sucked it up until this point. I had agreed, allowed that she knew best, so I took my leave.

Taking my leave meant walking back across the street where my fathers were, and maybe some of my mother's friends. I watched a nurse, tall, sturdy, German-looking, go to her side and tie her down to the gurney. She was to take her around the corner behind this rock and that would be it. She was about to roll the gurney to my mother's final moment, when I broke out of my submission and ran to her.

"Mom! Are you crazy? You can't do this!"

I hadn't seen if the nurse had already injected her with the deadly thing, but with everything in myself I moved back towards her, swearing that I would move time if I was too late.

What Not to Do

First, the pity face: mouth pursed, eyes squinched, "Ooh, I'm so sorryyyy ... well, good luck, dear." Aggravating. Who is that supposed to address? Certainly, not the person on the way to the hospital; more likely it's some sort of distancing guilt built on a secret whisper, "Glad that's not me."

Instead, the one reaction I appreciated came from a colleague, not even a close friend: "Congratulations on taking charge and taking care of your body. You'll do well."

A close second to the pity face is, "Does it hurt a lot?" or the variation, "You must be in great pain."

My answer is usually that I feel fine. Unless the person is a doctor, how is it their business what hurts and how badly? Actually, this seems like voyeurism to me, and though I've been polite, it occurred to me to answer, "No, I'm having back surgery for fun."

Then there was the well-meaning colleague who sincerely admonished me to chop off my fingernails and hair, leave all my cosmetics home, and find the ugliest over-sized baggy sweats to wear in order to set aside all thoughts of being attractive so that I would fully embrace the netherworld of the pitiable sick.

And finally, the old friend who visited from a distance and required attention – look what an effort he had made to see me! Like I was supposed to drop everything to soothe him, causing me to explain over and over what I was doing and why and reassure him when he asked what were the chances I was going to die.

Look, if you really care about somebody going to serious surgery, stow your fears and needs about yourself and say, "Good for you; you're going to be better."

The Metaphor

I never thought of myself as spineless or lacking in backbone, and if I've not always been straight up with people, that was for a purpose. I think I've maintained flexibility in my life, willingly, gladly embracing painting and book writing after my first profession as a screenwriter; I know I've been willing to bend to my daughter's talent as a musician. As for the metaphor of the spine so badly crooked, weak, and disintegrating that it's unable to support me or enable me to stand straight, none of that symbolism seems to fit.

Not that disease of any kind is caused by errors in life — a belief some people hold, superstitious in origin. And yet, yet, I do believe in a connection between mind and body so I wonder why has my central support, my spine gone astray? Have I betrayed myself, have I failed to stand up for myself? Should I never have married, never worked in teaching where my role was to support others to the point I could no longer carry them on my back, to the point they weighed me down? If so, will the steel rods give me a new will of steel? Is my courage going to be bolstered, and if so, who will I become?

May 13

≋

From Raya's Journal

My mom goes into the hospital in three days to get anterior and pos-
terior surgery on the lumbar region of her spine. She's getting a spinal
fusion to correct her scoliosis, steadied with two steel rods on either
side, screwed into her vertebrae, like Dr. Octopus from Spiderman Two
minus the sentient, evil, flailing arms. Worst of all, I find out just the
other day that she will NOT be able to receive HD transmissions or
satellite radio. Remind me again — what is the point of this?

These days I am trying to be peaceful, trying to be balanced to
support my mother. She is getting things in order around the house,
walking with her little teeter totter, making shopping lists for us, sche-
matics on the washer/dryer, getting bills in the mail so we won't be
naked and dirty while she's gone. She who spins our home on her
finger spins off so easily now, and I, dizzy artist, must assure the con-
tinued steady flow.

Inner peace is a type of insanity. It is a mindset made up of walls,
intentional blinders and denials just like other mindsets that are
regarded as less healthy. Inner peace is a contortion of reality com-
posed to channel one's thoughts in a particular direction. Albeit, this
state is better than others such as depression, anxiety, bi-polar, or "Star
Trek fan," still, it is just a mindset.

It is a glass plane that sits above a mess and a racket below. Or
maybe it's a plane of ice that melts when the one who sits upon it
becomes unwound and breaks a sweat. I believe this state of being
switches from being insanity to reality when doubt is gone. But there is
doubt like an imp on my shoulder, and fear strapped across my chest
— melting the foundation of my world.

May 14

≈

A Surrogate Mom

When I picture a first home in Los Angeles, I see the tiny house I rented on Third Street and Arnaz Drive, "Beverly Hills Adjacent," where I settled after college. At the time, from the mid-1970s through the early eighties, the area wasn't yet swanky. Behind my dollhouse spread a yard so generous I turned it into a farm and grew tomatoes, three kinds of squash, gigantic watermelons, corn, peas, beans, onions, and carrots surrounded by wild red, orange and yellow nasturtiums. My dear friend Martin, a free-living musician, parked his Econoline van in the driveway, a Ford with the end letters reversed to spell its name: Dorf. Eventually he and his guitar moved in and we married.

Those years sparkle in memory. Raya was born while we lived at that house. Among her early toys were round green peas from the garden that could be wonderfully discovered by unzipping the pod. And we had such a bumper crop of tomatoes we traded them to the restaurant next door in exchange for lunches.

Such a long time ago. Cedars-Sinai Medical Center was just being built on Third Street, commanding more real estate every year. The restaurant changed owners and became too uppity to buy our vegetables. And our dollhouse was sold to a company that covered the farmland with expensive condominiums.

After a while, Martin and I went separate ways, though he would always be one of my "immediate family." Of course, he'd wait with Raya and John at the hospital. It would be a few more years after moving from Arnaz Drive before I met and married

John. But this corner, exactly across from Cedars, would always be preserved in my memory at the moment when Raya was a beautiful child playing in a garden as tall as the sky above her, when everything was in bloom.

Martin and I had first met my friend Cathy when her baby and ours played in a nearby park, so Cathy knew the significance of this place when she chose to take Raya and me to a new restaurant on that same corner. Her goal was clear: Raya should regard her as a surrogate mom if I couldn't be around. Wisely, Cathy wanted to be a tangible presence, to hand Raya her phone number in person, to insist that Raya phone after each surgery, not because Cathy couldn't find the information by herself, but to stay in Raya's mind as a resource.

So there we stood, Cathy, Raya, and me on the very pavement squares where Raya learned to walk, now underneath the medical towers. The restaurant had become a favorite of entertainment executives on the hunt: young women in stiletto sandals, guys in Rolexes. In this context, I felt bent and shrunk even more, and I had no appetite. I was grateful as Cathy cheerfully handed her phone number to Raya and made small talk. But the concept of a surrogate mom so near "home" was too much for me, after all.

Finally, I just wanted to get on with the operation.

≈

From Raya's Journal

My mom, her friend Cathy and I had dinner at a restaurant called Barefoot. I haven't really reached into the significance of eating in my babyhood neighborhood with my mom so close to this major life crisis. I'm sure the meaning will surface, probably when I'm on the freeway, in the shower, or personally occupied with my boyfriend. He loves when I get inspired just before "the act." Yes, that's definitely his favorite.

Anyway, some meanings are obvious: the way some architecture changed and some didn't. Actually, most of the buildings on the street have changed, but the trees remained. The ballet studio was still there, the teepee-looking liquor store, the bakery — those have stayed while the rest of the area has been violently up-heaved.

And finally, my mother, still my mother, still green-eyed, tan and small — she was once again with me on this corner, standing with her daughter and her best friend. Here I was at a restaurant attached to a parking lot that I used to look down on from our second floor bathroom — and then over the top and across the street to the then still-growing Cedars-Sinai Hospital.

May 15

≈

From Raya's Journal

Morning prayer — first words in my head:

You can turn odds into evens,
You can turn love into sheer energy.

I'm aiming for miracles.
Help me make them easy.

Help me find sense
Like sipping from a stream.

The Night Before

The evening before surgery, John and I determined to go out to dinner, decidedly not deeming this a last supper. The household seemed to be holding its breath, as if a home could breathe. I'd put everything in place — a manual detailing everything from how to work the dishwasher to which bills might be urgent, but my instructions were limited to three weeks, as if that assured I'd return.

We'd carefully organized the next morning: John and Raya would take separate cars in case one needed to stay overnight, or if one needed a break, so someone would always be in the hospital, waiting for word. The clock would be set for 4 a.m. I'd pack right after dinner, but I already had my packing list. My email triggered an auto-response saying I wouldn't be answering until mid-June.

I wanted "clean" food tonight, aware my innards were unlikely to work for days or even weeks. In fact, I knew the surgeon was going to move my intestines around tomorrow ("within their sack," one of the doctors explained), as he accessed the front of my spine. That was just hours away. So we chose Real Food Daily, a vegan restaurant in Santa Monica, where everything is organic, dairy-free, close to raw and brimming with health. As if a mantra of scheduling could allay the possibility that something could go awry, we went over and over our simple plans.

But no sooner were we seated than something odd did occur, strange in a way that had nothing to do with all our planning. It reminded me that the visible plane on which we devise our lives is only that, like a graphic overlay beneath which are the actual circuits and energies that make things happen.

Now, this takes a little explaining. You know how sometimes you meet a person and instantly have a sense you know them, or once in a while you realize you have a deeper knowledge of someone's thoughts (actually more than thoughts — their *essence*), even if you know that person only superficially? Two people like that appeared in the past ten years, both friends of my daughter, so neither was a personal connection of mine. The first was a difficult young man my daughter had gone to school with; the second was Linda Martinez — more about her later.

As for this young man, I hadn't seen him in a long time, and he certainly wasn't on my mind as John and I sat down to dinner, when he appeared in the doorway. And, inevitably, the only available seat in the restaurant was beside me on the padded bench along a wall. I wondered whether or not to mention I was going to the hospital in the morning. But it came to me that the part of his soul that needed to know was not the person embodied in the seat next to me — if a meaning existed at all, it was happening on another level. Call it a past-life connection, or a vibration, or a different plane, somehow this spirit arrived at the restaurant serendipitously, as if he had to be present this one night to send me off, though I felt it was never necessary to say a word.

Later, John and I walked the length of the Santa Monica Promenade, promising that in a few months I'd be well enough to walk it again. He meant a victory stroll, but I slipped and called it a memorial walk. That stopped him cold. I corrected myself, of course. Really, I didn't think I was going to die, but the possibility hung in the air as we came home and asserted calm.

I packed and set my out-going phone message to say I was in the hospital. Then we brushed our teeth and quietly got into bed to wait for the morning.

May 15 — Night
≈

From Raya's Journal

I'm sure that when I bring her to the hospital, in my fear and my anxiety, despite my will to be calm and full of grace, my round moony eyes will be like two celestial jokes beneath an untamed cosmic disaster.

Maybe I'll listen to Billy Strayhorn's "Bloodcount" to get into the mood first. I'll groove my way into the surgical scene. I'll wear shades and something in leopard. Mom will like that.

≈

Affirmation

Thank you for making me strong and well, for straightening my back and helping me stand. Thank you for everywhere I'll walk, and for all I'll do in the years to come. Thank you for the wonderful success that will lead from this week and for all the hope it brings. Thank you for my days ahead when I'll dance.

Hospital
Days

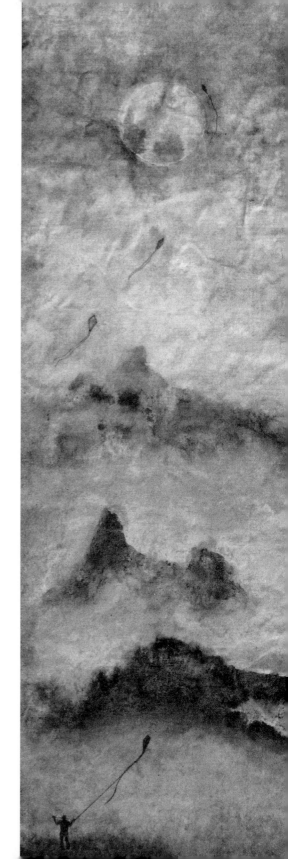

"I have always known
That I would take this road,
But yesterday
I did not know that it would be today."

— *Ariwara No Narihira, 9th Century Japan*

May 16

≈

Day One

Our radio-alarm burst into music at 4 a.m. as planned. John was first to take his shower and eat breakfast. At 4:15 Raya's alarm clock beeped and she took the second shower. I lay in bed, not really sleeping until 4:30. The third shower would be mine, careful to wash everywhere they might cut — not that they wouldn't disinfect me anyway. Of course I wasn't allowed to have breakfast. But in every other way, I followed my normal patterns — brushing my teeth, needlessly putting on a little makeup and dressing as I would for an ordinary day.

I packed my toothbrush and face creams, not so different from going on vacation, and oddly, I now realize, a few changes of clothes, and zipped the green tapestry suitcase. Long ago I'd named the suitcase "Fancy" because it wasn't like the serious black luggage that waited behind a door for some important flight to do business. No, Fancy, with its suggestions of perpetual flowering, had to come this day. I also took my journal though I never wrote a word. And I clutched my favorite handbag all the way into the pre-op room, making sure it was tight at my side even during the frightening days I was in the ICU.

It wasn't just any handbag. Linda Martinez had given it to Raya for her birthday, but it had quickly become mine. The bag had the style, originality and whimsy that reflected Linda, a camouflage pattern entirely in blues which would only camouflage someone who was in the sky, and a bold orange plastic handle which didn't pretend to match anything. The lining was furry and inside the bag was a change purse in the shape of a boy's underpants.

In my wallet were my essentials: my health insurance cards and driver's license, both necessary for admittance, and my non-essential testimonials to who I am: my membership in the Writers Guild of America, my USC faculty ID, a couple of video rental cards, my gym ID, and car insurance — evidence of a life in progress. My ATM card, cash, and keys couldn't come with me, I'd been warned, but I wasn't letting go of the rest.

Raya told me she'd been in touch with all the people and everyone was accounted for. I knew what she meant, but I sure didn't want to think about my parents who'd died a decade ago, not meaning to encourage a greeting party at the other side. Still, I must say I felt completely supported (not to indulge in hyperbole), and almost buoyed as if by pillows of air, the whole way there.

We left in two cars at exactly 5:00 before dawn. The streets were empty. Just before 5:30, we drove into the South Tower Parking for Cedars-Sinai Medical Center.

Cedars-Sinai — sometimes nicknamed Hotel Cedars or Gucci Center — is an impeccable host. Parking is located exactly at the entry for drop-off and pick-up, and is free those days, but pricey the rest of the time. At the registration desk, the security man had all my information right, and a volunteer immediately appeared to escort us to our floor. No question, we were already in their hands. So the three of us tramped to the elevators, to the 7th floor of the North Tower — Raya, carrying her laptop computer; John holding enough reading and design work to last a whole day, pulling Fancy; and me, clutching only Linda's bag and my journal.

We were seated in a reception lobby dotted with other people scheduled that morning. They seemed to come in twos, and I tried to guess which one was the patient, though I couldn't.

Nobody was talking. Raya opened her laptop to a file of photos we'd been in the midst of choosing for her new headshot, and we talked them over as if we had time to do this, all the while knowing that only minutes were available to tell her which one I thought was best.

A clerk was calling people to the side of a desk. I watched each go and come back to sit again in silence. Then they called my name. A well-organized man asked two questions that would be repeated many times that morning: What is your name, and why are you here today? Quickly, he took my insurance card and the referral that gave me a discount, and copied my driver's license. I signed some consents. Finally, he placed the plastic ID band on my right wrist. It wouldn't come off until I was home.

Now it was imminent, but we sat maybe ten minutes more as Raya and I kept discussing the photo file and John continued reading. At one end of the area, a large TV played CNN news headlines, though I doubt anyone was into it as they waited in silence.

Finally, a nurse appeared and read a list of eight names. One person in each party peeled away from a partner and assembled on line. I left Fancy in Raya's care — "Be sure to bring it to my room." But I never let go of the handbag. One glance back at Raya and John mutely watching me leave, and I turned away to walk, disappearing around a corner.

Next to me stood a tall, dignified African-American man with a resonant voice like James Earl Jones. As we walked, he said one sentence, "You are not alone."

In the pre-op room, each of us was ushered to a curtained bed; and each of us sat silently on the side of our bed, alone. The questions flew at me again, this time while checking my wrist bracelet: "What is your name? Why are you here today?" More consent forms to sign; then it moved quickly. I took off my clothes and shoes and put them along with Linda's handbag and the journal in white plastic bags — I wouldn't be dressed again for almost two weeks — and donned white pressure stockings and the first of many identical cotton hospital gowns I'd wear. Why anyone designed them with little squares in different shades of blue was a mystery. Surely a gown could look better, though, oddly, the sameness, the dullness, became almost comforting in the difficult days ahead.

More nurses, the anesthesiologist, and people whose jobs were mysterious crowded the bedside. An IV was started, taped to a vein inside my left elbow. The questions again: "What is your name? Why are you here today?" Efficient. In the next bed I overheard a man who spoke only Spanish, so his daughter stayed to translate. Then I met the most interesting of the medical team, a man whose entire practice was watching the surgery on a computer screen. He attached electrodes from my ankles all the way up my body. He'd monitor me continuously. I asked if he ever watched the actual surgery, but the question didn't make much sense: the electric paths of energy were the surgery, from his point of view.

And then there was nothing.

Monday, May 16

≈

From Raya's Journal

6:34 a.m.

Mom just went in. She was perky and positive, light on her feet. I heard a small string section in 3/4 time playing a happy chord, or maybe bittersweet, a major 6/9 chord, really very repetitive — Philip Glass in a good mood. It continued as she walked down the hall with the other people who were going to pre-op. The chord was fitting – bright, constant, like two in the afternoon.

When she turned the corner, the music persisted, but I felt a cold ball burst in my chest. She had turned around the canyon bend. The contents of the ball drained down the inside of me and now rest at my feet in a slight tingle. She looks so much younger than the others with her. Where is my other half going?

John and I are like new fish in a pet store floating around in a new bowl, completely unfamiliar with what we're seeing and experiencing. Little bubbles of conversation escape and go nowhere, bobbly eyes exploring different directions. All we want to see is her. All we can do is wait.

6:54 a.m.

Very inclined to run into the pre-op room, throw Mom over my shoulder and run out of the hospital "80's mad-cap comedy" style. I will bowl over doctors walking with notebooks, leap three feet ahead of me onto a gurney and sail down a hallway into a halfway closing elevator (at which point there will be an orchestrated hit denoting my incredible save). I am nuts. Maybe I'll watch the news.

7:00 a.m.

Why is there so much Lucite art in this hospital?

The First Surgery

(Michael Arango, Dr. Pashman's Private Surgical Technician, described my two surgeries, which are typical of this kind of procedure.)

Early in the morning, eight people surrounded my anaesthetized body lying prone on the operating table: the lead spine surgeon; a vascular surgeon; a third surgeon; a surgical technician; the anesthesiologist; a nurse; a nerve conduction technician; an X-ray technician; and a cell saver to recycle my blood.

The vascular surgeon made the first cut on my left flank from the side of my abdomen all the way around to my back; it's called a thoracic abdominal incision. This was to expose the rib which would be cut and also the front of my spine.

The surgeons then cut through the peritoneum, which is the lining that covers most abdominal organs, and stripped all the muscles off my 11th rib at the bottom of my rib cage. The surgeon lifted the rib, separating it from the inside organs. With a bone cutter, which is like a small shear, the rib bone was cut.

Going behind the sac that holds the internal organs, the entire bag was moved aside to expose the spine. Once the spine was exposed, they took a fluoroscopic picture, which is a kind of X-ray, to verify they were at the correct level of the spine. Then Dr. Pashman took over.

He cut into the spine to take out the discs. Using a special instrument like a kind of pliers, he bit out four or five discs, which are a rubbery material that separate the vertebrae, from

T12 to L5 (from my mid-back to the bottom of my lower back). With the discs gone, my spine released to straighten somewhat.

Meanwhile, the rib was ground down to a powder in a bone mill. This powder was packed into the space where the discs were removed to cause a fusion.

Earlier when they reached into my chest to get to the 12th level, they had to breach my diaphragm; that collapsed my left lung, a common occurrence. So on closing, they inserted a chest tube which sucked out pressure, creating a negative space to make the lung re-inflate. Finally, the bag with my internal organs was set back in place, and they sewed me up.

May 16

≈

After the First Surgery

Later, I learned that Martin arrived and sat in the waiting area with John and Raya for hours.

From the scars, I could tell they'd cut from my left side all the way around to my back, but my abdominal muscles remained intact — I'd specifically chosen the side cut and I think it helped me walk as soon as I did. An alternate route to the front of my spine might have been a keyhole cut around my navel, then vertically south down my belly. Awfully glad that didn't happen.

Whatever they did in there turned out more painful than the larger surgery on my back two days later; it took weeks for that searing side pain to subside. And whatever they did with my intestines remained a challenge more than a month later — they worked, but not as easily at first.

Meanwhile, John and Raya and Martin waited. Doctors came out and reported to other families, but the hours went by and no one came about me. Finally the receptionist's phone rang and she asked for John. He told me that he stood and counted the thirty paces to the desk wondering why he was being called; why did no one come out? On the phone, Dr. Pashman said the operation went well, and they were closing. And that was that.

I don't remember, but I'm told the three of them saw me in my room. Those early days were a blur of pain meds and sleep, so I have only a vague image of all three faces attempting to smile at me while a plastic tube sprayed oxygen into my nose, a catheter collected urine into a rectangular plastic container, and IV tubes hung everywhere.

An epidural implanted directly near my spine released a narcotic each time I pressed a button (and I do recall pressing it often though I don't actually remember the pain). I did have the presence of mind to ask for nausea meds even before I needed them because, once in the past, I'd became nauseated from anesthesia and I wasn't taking a chance. I remember being thirsty, though the nurses couldn't let me have water.

It seemed impossible that I would go through this all over again in just two days, but I was on the train now, and there was no getting off.

May 17

≈

Day Two

In the day between surgeries, nurse Maddy urged me out of bed, her arms spread as if to waltz, encouraging me to breathe, "Smell the roses, blow out the candles." Thus we danced, me a wreck in my hospital gown, barely able to move (certainly not able to stand or walk by myself) and she, a sturdy middle-aged woman with an Armenian accent.

The notion that I could get out of bed at all seemed bizarre. First, my left side — the site of the incision — seared like a hot blade every time I leaned, making it next to impossible to bend to sit up from the bed. The hospital beds are so high that my feet were miles from the floor as Maddy tried to talk me down. Somehow, she prevailed, with me draped around her rather than really walking, and she sat me in a chair. There I stayed rigid, unmoving, staring blankly at the TV until rescued back into bed an hour later. Throughout, I was lucid enough to know I looked lousy and to decide I didn't care.

Another nurse said every day I'd feel a little better. But I told her that the second, larger operation was tomorrow. Her mouth formed an "ooh" and she said no more.

≈

The Second Surgery

Anaesthetized, I was placed face down with my hands angled at ninety degrees from my shoulders, and elbows bent, like someone flying.

This was the larger surgery to place steel rods down my entire back, and it required a very long incision. Dr. Pashman worked slowly, cauterizing (burning to stop bleeding) immediately after each small cut. The blade went through skin then fatty tissue and finally muscles.

With retractors he spread the muscles and dissected the tissues away from the spine, cutting all the meat from the bone. The dissection was slow and meticulous until the spine was completely clear.

Some of the bone was also shaved to enable the spine to flex. That bone was collected and powdered for use later.

Now Dr. Pashman began the steps to place metal screws into the pedicles of the spine (pedicles are like spokes around the spinal cord). Using X-rays, a microscope and micro-instruments, he verified the precise locations on the pedicles to place the screws.

With a special kind of screwdriver, twelve large screws went into the bone. Each has a head into which the rods fit, somewhat like guiding train tracks.

Then Dr. Pashman bent the steel rods with a rod bender because after a lifetime a curved spine couldn't straighten completely. Once the rods were in, the bone that had been shaved was put back on the spine, especially at the apex of the curve and at the bottom so it would fuse and add strength.

From the first preparations until closing, I was unconscious in the operating room for about eight hours.

May 18

≈

After the Second Surgery

I remember, only vaguely, a night-shift nurse murmuring, "You're going to surgery now," in the wee hours of May 18th. Unlike the first operation, I was knocked out while they prepped me. No one asked my name or why I was there anymore.

I'd been told what they were going to do: turn me over, propped on some sort of blocks, and the team would insert the metal rods on each side of my spine that had been fused two days before. Later, X-rays showed me how extensive this procedure actually was. In addition to the vertical steel rods, I had an array of what looked like long nails from a side view, forming a kind of arc around my tail bone, and screws attached to the vertebrae.

Meanwhile, Raya, John and Martin took up residence in my room in the afternoon, expecting me to be wheeled back at any moment. They had dinner, then they watched an episode of "Lost," which ran from 8 to 9 p.m. Still, I hadn't come back. A security guard told them visiting hours were over and they'd have to get a pass to stay. More than eight hours had passed since I'd entered the operating room and no one knew where I was or what had happened.

It's normal for a patient to go to a recovery room after surgery. My family knew that, but they figured sooner or later I'd be wheeled in, as I had been after the first surgery. Now it was around twelve hours after I'd been taken to surgery. This time, I couldn't return at all. Nurses were working on me as my blood pressure rose and fell precipitously. Finally, they consigned me to the Intensive Care Unit, where I would stay for four days.

Later, Raya told me she finally learned from a nurse that I wasn't coming back to the room; I'd been taken to the ICU. A hot shock ran through her body and she steeled herself. As John and Martin went for the passes, Raya slipped down the hall in search of the ICU, wherever that might be. She wandered, then followed the signs, determined to find her mother and see that I was alive.

She rang the bell to the locked ICU. A nurse let her in and led her to an alarming sight: I was drained of color; my belly had ballooned like a beach ball; my lips were puffy and my eyes so swollen they couldn't open. I was moaning. But I was alive. It turned out I'd lost so much blood I needed a transfusion of the blood I'd banked. Thank goodness I had donated two pints because I received one that first day and the second pint the next day. My eyes felt crusted shut and my mouth was parched. I asked for water but a nurse said I could only have a piece of ice. I whispered that ice was too cold, and Raya said she was over-joyed: if I could complain I was still me.

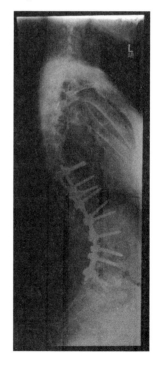

Vaguely, I could see I was in an industrial sort of cubicle stocked with machines, especially a heart monitor that beeped all the time. Raya told me she stared at the numbers, especially when they escalated and the green digits changed to red, no doubt a warn-ing, but no one would explain what they meant. By the next day, a blister would appear on my distended chin, probably a result of lying face down for hours.

Thus, I fell asleep, and the operation was deemed a success.

May 18

≈

From Raya's Journal

You know, it just hit me. Today, a team of men knocked my mother out and hurt her in some of the most pre-meditated, severe, dangerous and creative ways yet conceived. I told my boyfriend last night, "Because they're doctors they can do this. If anyone else had hurt her like that, I'd kill them." No response from boyfriend.

I saw her in the ICU for the first time after the last operation. Her face, all of her, was so swollen, so colorless, she barely looked real. There were purple spots on her tongue, her middle looked impregnated, and her face seemed to be inflated. This was all apparently due to some substantial blood loss. However, I saw her eyes. This was how I knew it was her. The shape of her face was stretched as if someone had painted it and rolled it from side to side on a flat cloth and held the picture up. Her eyes were puffed shut, but still, when she realized I was there she looked at me, and I saw the emeralds. Within this yellowed flesh gorged with fluid, she managed to open her lids enough to see me, and enough for the green lightning to flash me her spirit, still there under everything. A moment later a nurse adjusted her and she complained. It was music to my ears.

Martin's Reactions

Hospitals have a certain vibration that I associate with a smell. It brought up uneasy feelings as I walked into the waiting room and saw Raya and John sitting with their backs to the window. Right away, Raya hugged me. She's very strong and doesn't want to show how she feels, so I tried not to talk about what was happening, but when we did I made sure it was always upbeat.

By one in the afternoon, John had already heard from the doctor that they were closing and he brought me up-to-date. Pam had been in there a long time by then. A lot of things go through your mind, like how long can they hold a body open. I'd never had a serious operation like that, so I didn't have much data on how Pam might feel. We just focused on what a good mood she was projecting as she got ready for it.

When I saw her in the bed, I thought how tender things were at that moment. I remembered when we lived in the house on Third Street when she first began jogging. We used to go over to the school before it opened in the morning and run around the track. She didn't think she could do it at first, but after some heavy persuasion I got her jogging and she took right to it as soon as she had somebody believing in her. After that, she did a lot of jogging and I was proud of her. So I thought, well, she can do it again. I tried to bring forward what I'd felt back then, bring what she'd achieved into that moment, and hold that image there, put that vibration in the room. I closed my eyes and meditated, seeing her well. That's all you can do.

For the second operation, we were waiting in the room, expecting Pam to be brought back, but they kept giving us excuses why we couldn't see her, and I thought, oh this doesn't look good. So Raya and I held hands. The nurses were saying she was probably in the recovery room, but they didn't give any indication that anything was up with her.

Finally at 9 p.m. the security guard came up to us and said we had to leave, so we went downstairs and got the bracelets from security so we could stay. It was kind of scary because they didn't want to tell us where Pam was. I have to admit it was a little touch and go there; my wall started to crumble a little bit and sneak over to the negative which was where I didn't want to go.

Finally we went into the ICU room, all of us. The room was full of machines and buzzes and whirls and all kinds of sounds and people in strange outfits. It really bothered me to see Pam like that. She was puffed up and she didn't look like herself. They had to take stuff out of her belly to get to what they wanted, then put it back, so she was all bloated. My mind didn't have answers for all of that so I just kind of "ducked and covered" mentally.

Pam kept saying, "Leave, go, I'll be okay."

It hurt a lot to see her that way. Her color was weird, her face was puffy. I imagined the emergency workroom in her body going crazy — we need blood over here, send supplies over there. All we could do was send our love and back off. That's all we could do. I went home and thought a lot about her, meditated, lit a candle.

When things like that happen to people who are that close, life really comes into focus. You think about yourself, you think about them: What are you going to do if they're gone? What if you're gone? Did I say the right things? I worried about adjusting to life if something happened. Could I step up to the plate? Did I say enough things to her? Did I say enough things to Raya?

You start worrying about the people around you, rather than yourself: How are they going to be if the world you knew, and know, is changing? You think about that. The only thing you can do is keep on keeping on. You do the best you can, enjoy what you had and have, and keep on going.

The ICU

The next three days were like a single unending day in the permanent hard light of the Intensive Care Unit. The door to my cubicle — a space that could fit only my bed and the hospital machines — had to remain open so the heart monitor could be viewed from the nurse's station. Doctors came and went. Nurses checked me often, but I was too drugged to keep track.

Apparently, my blood pressure had descended precipitously and my heart started struggling. Raya said she could actually see it pumping and each heartbeat shook my entire body. Someone thought this was caused by the implanted epidural which delivered morphine directly to my back, and removed it. I later heard that my main surgeon hadn't agreed. I don't know. Honestly, I was never afraid; I knew I'd get past this phase.

It was an interesting, active scene. Cheryl, my night nurse, was pregnant, working only three more weeks until her maternity leave. On her feet for 15-hour shifts, she claimed she didn't mind, since full-time consisted of three 15-hour days per week, which gave her four days off. Here she was, about to have her first child, yet she confided that what really worried her was her mother arriving from out of town, and moving in for a month after the baby is born. With all the life and death around her, Cheryl was anxious only that her mom would criticize her if the house wasn't perfectly clean and in order.

I met Jason, another nurse, an ambitious young man, the only white male nurse I'd encountered out of a dozen or so nurses throughout my stay. He wanted me to know that he'd gone through four years of a rigorous college program to get his nursing degree, and that he was taking advanced classes to be an anesthesiology nurse.

Then there was the young doctor (not one of my regulars) who came to check my heart at a particularly inauspicious time when I'd wet the bedding. I looked like a whale and probably smelled like one too. He read my chart and discovered I was a screenwriter, so he pitched, "I have some great ideas for movies." Sounds like a joke, but this is L.A. I dryly remarked "I don't think this is a good time," and he muttered reluctantly, "Oh, yeah."

Some cubicles down, a man kept screaming "Help! Help!" The nurses didn't react; I discovered he'd screamed until he was moved the next day. They were consummate professionals, every one of the staff, and I had absolute confidence in their care. But despite their skills, ICU patients sometimes didn't make it. One time I woke up to overhear the nurses discussing the time a Code Blue was called, and the time of death. I asked if someone had died, and was only told that it was "someone who was very, very sick." They carefully revealed no more. Yes, people died all the time where I was.

Codes came in other colors. Once I heard a Code Red, which I found out meant smoke (check for fire). And long after I was out of the ICU, a Code Green sounded in the corridor: a child had escaped down on the third floor and was running around the halls.

Ever present in the ICU were the giants in blue, men and women with muscles of weight-lifters wearing blue overalls with wide leather back supports, whose job was to lift people and move them. From the number of times I saw the body-builders, a whole lot of heavy people in the ICU must have needed carrying.

In time, my heart adjusted itself, my blood pressure normalized, and though I still couldn't get out of bed (in the ICU they don't even try, nor could they, not with all the delicate hook-ups in the way), I'd survived the steel and glass intensive care, and I would be moved to a real room.

May 21

≈

Traveling

In normal life, we move where we must. In charge of our bodies, we decide to turn left, to open a door, or change our minds and not go at all. As a hospital patient, that essential volition, that power over your own choices, over where you'll be, is surrendered.

Most of the beds, it seemed, are interchangeable, so attendants prop up the metal bars on the sides of the bed, release the brake, and transport you along with the entire bed. But sometimes you need to be transferred to a gurney, so another bed is brought and lined up next to yours. Then the body builders lift the sheet that you're on, one muscled pair of arms at your head, the other at your feet, and slide you (with your sheet) to the gurney. They're good at it, but if anything is fragile or delicately held at bay, no movement is gentle enough. And, of course, they have to tug you back into a bed when you arrive.

On the day I left the ICU, I asked the "movers" to make sure they took my worldly possessions: Fancy, the carefully-packed suitcase, not opened since I arrived; the two white plastic bags marked "patient property" with my clothes and shoes that I'd worn to the hospital at 5:00 a.m. on May 16; and I clutched Linda's handbag to my side under a top sheet.

My friend Ellen had brought me some books, but in the move they were left behind. I never did find them. I was told people had sent bouquets, but flowers aren't allowed in the ICU, so to this day I don't know where they went or whom to thank.

Traveling on a bed through the hallways reduces you to an object of curiosity, an object lesson: Don't get sick like that. Mostly the corridors are empty or lined with health-workers who are unfazed. But the elevator is public and large enough for a bed. I'm wheeled in, lying next to civilians in their street clothes, busy on their cell phones, laughing together, careful not to make eye-contact with the "other," the one whose hair is unkempt, face unattended, horizontal in the center of the space.

At last, I was relieved to have it over with as we approached Room 8110 on the glorious 8th floor.

May 19-21

From Raya's Journal

On May 19th, the first full day my mother is in the ICU, I am up in the morning, checking my email. The lyrics to the Paul Simon song "Call Me Al" pop into my head. For some reason, the lyrics are sticking to me, and I am moved to sing them out loud. I sing them slow, loud, soft, whispered, nearly spoken:

"A man walks down the street, he's in a strange world, maybe it's the third world, maybe it's his first time around...."

I go outside and sit on the grass. I sing the lyric in the first person, "Maybe it's my first time around...." I look up at the tangerine tree and the spindly orange tree which still manages two miraculous oranges.

"He sees angels in the architecture. He says hallelujah, hallelujah."

I sing all this with my heart up to the new day and this new world of faith and chance in which I find myself. My vision has been clarified and simultaneously dumbfounded by the matter-of-fact way that drastic changes take place. A breeze passes over me and I try to smell what God is cooking.

Then a particular phrase came out of the song and took me by the shoulders:

"Who will be my role model now that my role model is gone?"

This moment in the song aches through me involuntarily. For some reason these words seem to be the most true expression at this moment. I repeat them many times.

That night at around 2 a.m. I get a phone call. It is very late so I hope it isn't the hospital telling me that my mother has taken a bad turn, I look at the cell phone screen and I see that it is my friend Steve, a bass player I have known since college.

"Raya, something terrible has happened."

I cannot imagine what. He doesn't even know my mom, and that is the core drama in my life at the moment. What else could possibly matter?

"What happened?"

"Linda. She killed herself. She did it today. She's gone."

The shock was transformative. Every task of mine completed that day shrank into miniatures on a model train set shadowed by the cloud of this loss. Linda? My music sister, the one who looks more like my family than I do, the one who taught me how to pluck my eyebrows, fake my ID, who showed me what the hell a I-VI-ii-V chord progression was. I sat on the bed with nothing. I had nothing to say to anyone, nothing to say to myself. All I had was the song, still cycling through my mind, getting stuck on that phrase:

"Who will be my role model now that my role model is gone?"

Linda

I recognized Linda Martinez as a sort of soul reflection from the first time I met her in 1997. My daughter was in high school; Linda had graduated from college and was already a successful pianist, composing and later touring with "Destiny's Child," and writing music for movies and TV shows. When she was 15 she'd won the "Spotlight Award" given to young artists by the Los Angeles Music Center, and years later when Raya competed, the Spotlight director put the girls together on radio shows and performances where Linda was a kind of mentor.

But none of that mattered ultimately. Linda looked somewhat like me, and when the three of us — Linda, Raya and I — stood together, we were sometimes asked if we all were sisters (a compliment to me of course), and with straight faces we answered "yes" more than not. About a year ago when Raya and I highlighted our dark hair, Raya commented we wouldn't look like Linda anymore. But a week later when we saw Linda, we discovered she had highlighted her hair at the same time. A mere coincidence, of course, and yet you wonder about the consonance of energies.

Lately, Linda had become thin. A couple of years earlier, her father, whom she adored, died of cancer after a long struggle. I remembered seeing her climb into the audience after she and Raya had performed with a band at the Hollywood Bowl — watching Linda sit on those hard bleachers next to her dad, holding his hand, and how proud of her he was. She missed him.

The last time I saw Linda (a few weeks before I'd entered the hospital), at one of Raya's shows, we'd hugged, as always, and her shoulders seemed frail. She'd spent the entire show standing because it hurt too much to sit ever since she'd developed a disc problem in her back. That must have been awful for a pianist, not to be able to sit without pain. She asked about my upcoming surgery and I told her I'd email her my doctor's phone number, though I wanted to see how well I'd come out before I recommended this to anyone. Then in the week before my surgery, Raya had several lunch dates with Linda made and cancelled because everyone was too busy.

On March 19, the day after my main surgery, Raya's phone rang at 2 a.m. Raya told me she'd felt an awful premonition: who would be calling at two in the morning? No, it wasn't about me; I wasn't in danger. It was a friend saying Linda was dead. She'd committed suicide by overdosing on prescription sleeping pills. In the weeks after, everyone tried to understand. She'd sometimes spoken of the music that she could never turn off in her head, and she'd been on anti-depressants, but none of those explanations sufficed.

While I was in the ICU, Raya didn't tell me. One day, the following week, she came from the funeral wearing a black jacket that Linda had given her years ago. Raya only said that she'd been at an event. I'd felt no "disturbance in the force," though I was in too much of a disturbance myself to be aware of anything else. Not until I was packed to come home did she tell me.

After the shock, what resonated was the vast mystery of balance in the universe: I, who might have died, was going home. Linda was dead at 29. Rationally, any connection makes no sense, but as I left the hospital I had the same glimpse of wholeness, of larger rhythms, of being within vibrations that I'd had when I'd arrived unafraid that first dawn. And somehow, within all that, maybe Linda had completed what she was here to do. It was for us to behold in awe.

Hotel Cedars

After the ICU, Room 8110 seemed palatial. As I was wheeled through the large door, the suite opened to a "living room" on the left with a full couch, a round dining table and upholstered chairs. Behind the table, a picture window viewed the Hollywood Hills rolling clear back to a perfect blue sky, high enough above traffic to frame only the idyllic landscape.

In the center, an array of doors opened to the bathroom area, a large double sink flanked by separate rooms for the shower and commode. The faucets were bordered in gold.

On the right, my bed was settled against an impressive wooden headboard that subsumed the ports for equipment in its carvings. A tall well-cushioned armchair faced the second picture window where construction of a new wing blocked some of the view; but from the chair, a green avenue of trees led up to the hills. Every night, star-points of lights from the houses in the hills winked that the world did exist beyond these walls.

As my bed, IV, and all the other instruments were plugged in, I gazed at the fine, large Georgia O'Keefe print on the right wall and determined to be able to get up and look at the art on the other walls one day. Soon the nurses left me. I turned on the ceiling-mounted TV. This would be home for a while.

The eighth floor was for high-ticket surgeries, and probably high-ticket patients. The hallways had been curated (rather than decorated) by someone with sophisticated taste. The nurses didn't like the art, but I was tickled to think I'd been placed in a fine art gallery to get well.

If someone paid for a spine fusion like mine without insurance, and the preferred-provider discounts and the in-network referrals that I was fortunate to have, the sticker price might be as high as half a million dollars once the weeks at Hotel Cedars were tallied. Thanks to the wonderful Writers Guild Health Fund (a group insurance plan available to members of the Writers Guild of America), combined with using in-network pre-approved services through the Motion Picture Television Fund, and their negotiated arrangements with Blue Cross, I was elevated to eighth floor status without paying hundreds of thousands.

I later discovered that this floor was special in other ways. On the usual hall chart listing patients, doctors and room numbers, patient names had been expunged, and a sign was posted on at least one door: "name security." I guessed a celebrity was in there. The nurses and nurse's aids (titled "Clinical Associates" here) were unimpressed.

As one of them put it, "A body is a body, doesn't matter if man or woman or who; everyone is the same — a body."

Despite the luxury of this suite, my reality was that I could barely move. My body was still swollen, my left side shot a pain from my ribs down my legs if I so much as turned, and I couldn't eat. Nor did I have the energy — the drive — to do anything else, not even read a book, certainly not to write, as I lay in the same position in bed day after day.

Then early one morning I woke to see men rappelling down the construction wall out the window. They had lowered ropes and scaffolding. On the roof, men were turning a pulley as the climbers in hard hats balanced on ledges. Reaching out from the ledges, they tore off immense sheets of plastic and dropped them out of sight far below, unwrapping the wall like a giant gift box. As I watched them it became clear: All this waiting, lying still, was because I was under construction too, and one day I would be unwrapped to reveal a shiny structure, tall and new, reflecting the early sun.

Visits

The days had a predictable rhythm, one indistinguishable one from the next, except that mornings were signaled by a flurry of specialists, and nights by a nurse turning off the lights, probably more to relieve the tired night shift than for patients like me who'd slept most of the day. Night was defined mostly by being lonely — even frightening — confined to a bed from which I couldn't escape, knowing hours might pass before anyone came.

I got to know the night nurses; they had to stay awake too, without much happening. Day and night, the nursing staff could have sung "We Are the World," mostly young women from Asian, South Pacific, former-Soviet, and Latin American countries, and some African-Americans.

I still liked Maddie especially, who danced me out of bed when no one else could, holding me up and encouraging me to breathe: "Smell the roses, blow out the candles."

That was better than the nurse whose voice trembled with alarm as she warned, "Keep your eyes open or you're going to faint!" knowing she wasn't big enough to break my fall or pick me up.

Another favorite confided that she was only on a month-to-month contract because she had to be free to go to science fiction conventions. Most of them spoke to me like I might be a person with the ideas that used to interest me; they reminded me that I would be engaged in something outside that room again.

Pushing a call button floated a disembodied voice into the room: "Yes?" I'd say it's time for my pain pills, or I need help sitting (or, when I was better, help getting up from the chair or the commode). Soon one of my new friends would appear. It was a lifeline, that button, and the times it fell off the bed into the unreachable abyss below, I lay helpless, bereft.

At the end of the night shift, the nurses convened at a staff meeting which created a palpable void before the morning storm. The visits began at 7 a.m. with the Doctor of Internal Medicine who was also the respiratory specialist. One of my lungs had collapsed in surgery (a common occurrence, I'm told), so I was supposed to be sucking and blowing into a little plastic device that held three blue balls. The object was to make all three balls rise, but with the entirety of my wind power the first ball bobbled near the bottom.

"You're supposed to do that once every ten minutes, and cough to get the gunk out of the bottom of your lungs," he admonished.

Yeah, right. I was asleep every ten minutes, and coughing? You gotta be kidding; why would I rattle the particles that screamed every time I moved. But it was this doctor's job to persuade me to take impossible breaths into a chest that ached, and somehow ingest acrid potassium pills sized for livestock. (I did discover that breaking them into tiny bits mixed in apple sauce helped.) He was a good doctor. I know because I survived.

Second in the parade was a woman from the cardiac department — not to be asked about pills or anything else, she informed me. All day, nurses took my blood pressure, and placed my index finger in a device that somehow measured the oxygen in my blood. But she also pricked my finger and checked some other numbers before wheeling her equipment cart to the next room without a sign of what it all meant.

Then came one of Dr. Pashman's fellows (doctors who are learning a specialty; they seem to rotate every few months or so). The process made me think of plant propagation, like Johnny Appleseed spreading apple trees throughout the West. These guys were going to be cutting someone's back miles away one day — hundreds of thousands of spines on earth fused and held up by steel rods. What does that suggest about the human condition as bipeds?

In any case, the young doctor looked briefly at the scar and pronounced it okay, squeezed my ankles to make sure they hadn't turned to cottage cheese, and asked me to push against his hand with my right foot, then left foot. Finally, he asked how I was doing, which he could see for himself as I lay there looking like a walrus. Thinking all was fine, he departed.

On his heels, a marvel of logistics arrived: the breakfast tray. The friendly server, who was not supposed to touch the patient or the bed, had two choices: (1) put the tray on a table that might as well be in the next state for someone unable to get there, or (2) set it on a rolling table that slid across the bed. This works only theoretically. If you're six feet tall, you could push the button to angle the bed to sitting so you could reach the tray. For me, I was stuck lying underneath it, staring up at the bottom of food, since the only thing the bed would tilt was the pillow above my scalp. I pressed the call button, and eventually someone strong would do the sheet-pull to lift me way to the top and sit me up partially.

By the end of the week, I was asking nurses to put me in a chair, so the breakfast challenge was won, at least geographically, though it would be weeks before I really began to eat. Nevertheless, in a fit of optimism, I filled out my menu for the next day. In those early days I relished my only adult task: I'd read words and write down an opinion.

Usually the rehabilitation specialist showed up just as I attempted my first sip of coffee. These athletic women, bright-eyed and eager to get people moving, went from one room to the next, and if you weren't ready you lost your turn. I'd hoped they might have done some of the exercises I'd learned in Pilates or Yoga, or even a version of muscle-building I'd seen at the gym, or maybe some movements designed for the bed-ridden. But at this stage, the goal was only to get up and "walk." In my case, walking consisted of leaning on a square gray metal walker (like I'd seen very old people use) and trying to make my legs step forward.

The first time I reached the round table at the far window in my room — ten steps exactly — felt like completing a marathon; there should have been a ribbon. The best day was when I exceeded the boundary of my room and stepped into the corridor, and then crossed it to touch the opposite wall. After that, I gradually walked the halls with the rehab person every day, tethered to her with a kind of leash in case I fell. Oh well, I kept my eyes on the fine art that lined the route, and I peeked into the open rooms, wondering if the haggard faces who looked out were able to leave their confinement.

But those victories didn't come until the last few days. One of the early mornings in Room 8110, I remember promising myself: Today I'm going to get up and I'll stand by myself, and then I'll start walking, and go past my door, and down the first corridor, around the corner, and, by then, I'll be walking faster, and I'll make the entire circle around the floor before coming back and sitting in a chair instead of lying in bed. That day when the rehab person came, I did get out of bed. I stood up. But before I took a single step, I was overwhelmed by weakness, so dizzying, I might have fainted. I was breathing hard when they put me back in bed.

I begged, "Please come back; I'll try again later."

But the rehab specialist didn't return that day. I'd used up my chance.

After "rehab" came the Occupational Therapist. Understand, my occupations are writing and painting. Could she improve my computer's spell-check feature, or schedule a gallery show? It turned out that the OCT addressed practical tasks of daily life, so if your "occupation" was using the toilet, they had suggestions. Actually, this is serious. After back surgery, you can't bend, twist, lift anything, or stand up from a chair, not to mention being unable to walk anywhere. If you're also wearing a huge, bulky brace, as I was, and you're not an orangutan, you have no way of reaching beyond the brace under your hips. Think about that.

All those specialists lined up at my bedside from the moment I woke until nearly lunch. I had no time to brush my teeth, wash my face, fix my hair, eat, or clean up in any way. So when the nurse appeared with my next batch of meds, I asked for one of the most valuable items I brought to the hospital:

OLAY Daily Facials Express Wet Cleansing Cloths — "no water needed."

I'm so glad I thought of that in advance. Like any quality lodging, "Hotel Cedars" provided amenities to each guest: travel sizes of skin lotions, shampoo, conditioner, toothbrushes, toothpaste, mouthwash, facial cleansers, body powders, washcloths, and so forth. They were like siren calls from distant shores. Stuck in bed, you need your own survival kit. For me, two packages of those Olay wet-wipes, a compact mirror, and a few cosmetics I carried in my handbag put me in charge of my face at least, though the rest of me stayed funky. During my twelve days in the hospital, I was washed only three times, once in the ICU and two showers in the days before I came home. It seems this kind of personal care is up to the patient. Be prepared.

I really didn't want visitors. Still, two friends showed up uninvited, and after exclaiming, "You look great!" (I looked terrible so I wondered how much worse they'd expected), they sat awkwardly on the edge of the chairs for maybe fifteen minutes and couldn't wait to get out of there. No one really wants to visit a hospital; it was kind of them to give it a try.

But visits from my family were sweet; they brought their dinners and sat with me as I pretended to eat. John watched TV at my side, almost like home. I still see Martin's wistful eyes as he recalled being with me in the hospital when Raya was born, as fresh a memory as if it were today. Raya took care to wear cheerful colors (except the day of Linda's funeral) and looked like an angel bouncing into my room with her gold-tinged curls. One day she brought her guitar and sang to me. Those visits to Room 8110 were precious.

≈

Bedpans

Human beings can adjust to circumstances that would otherwise be unthinkable indignities, setting a new standard of acceptable behavior with an ease that suggests how the species adapted to survive. In a hospital, no bodily process is private — they are merely functions of an organism. And you, the patient, must accept, even embrace, being that shared organism if you're going to survive like the cave people, nomad and hunter-gatherers did before.

With that philosophical shield, I peed into a pot. Not quite that simple. Maybe men have it easy when the nurse holds up an index finger and asks "Number one?" But a woman who is bed-ridden — that is, who can't possibly get to a commode (not even a portable one three feet from the bed) — requires gymnastics, courage, and the willingness to rely on mercy.

The last is not really in your control. Nurse's aides (who may resent this job to varying degrees) have to bring over the bedpan, a gray plastic oval. Somehow you need to roll on your side as it arrives. I gripped the metal bars on the bedside and pulled myself over on one hip to the extent I could, no matter how much that hurt. Then, hanging on to those bars with all my might, I'd wait for the aide to slide the pan under me. Once it was there, I could roll back over the hard plastic. Considerate nurses would come back in a couple of minutes. Others had to be called.

The mental challenge — overriding your childhood admonitions not to wet the bed — is to let go. You don't really have a choice anyway, but the first time it's difficult to escape the sense you've done something wrong, and the notion that the sheets are drenched.

To get the bedpan away requires the same strength, rolling to the side, gripping metal. You have to cling in that position until the aide cleans you off. The professionals squirt a little cleansing water and might even dust some powder, like tending a baby. But most give a few dabs with a wash cloth, leaving you not so "fresh" as they say in the commercials.

At least the physical ordeal is over after that. You can roll onto your back and sleep — until the next time. If your body is flushing out the drugs (especially the anesthesia, which seems to linger in the system a while) and you have a continuous IV drip hydrating you, you'll be asking for that bedpan every few hours.

What you find out — what I discovered anyway — is that you don't need to hide from those helpers, or avoid letting them know you as a person. For the best of them, bringing and taking a bedpan isn't so different from changing your IV or helping you stand. I said "Thank you" each time, and talked to those who wanted to be friendly. By not identifying yourself as embarrassed, the process falls into perspective as one small aspect of healing.

Then get the heck out of that bed as soon as you can.

The Braceman Cometh

While I still lay like a bloated sea mammal beached helplessly on the bed, a young man from Lerman, the brace company, appeared. He was going to measure me for a "custom" brace, made to fit perfectly around the aforementioned beach ball.

Given that I couldn't lean or turn, when he explained he planned to wrap me in a plaster cast, I said, "You gotta be kidding." But he had no sense of humor. The first step was spanning my pubic bone to my collar bone with a tape measure, circling the balloon, and writing some numbers on a pad. Then he proceeded to the plaster. This involved removing my gown and laying wet strips over me which dried into plaster surprisingly quickly.

As for turning me over on my stomach, that took two people. I remember that it hurt, but one strange quality of pain is that the brain doesn't seem to retain the sensation, only the fact that it had existed, as if it were someone else's experience. Maybe that's an evolutionary protection for survival, I don't know. I vaguely recall hollering, and that soon it was over. They were gone and I was left dusted with white plaster like beach sand.

The next day he was back with a brace so heavy I couldn't lift it, and so humongous I couldn't lower my arms or my chin when I tried it on. I also insisted they make holes throughout the plaster so it would breathe in the coming summer. Two days later, he returned with a trimmed down version which I endured until a month after I was home from the hospital. That's when I went to the main office and had it re-fitted, cut down entirely.

As weak as I felt, I wasn't going to stand by (okay, lie by) and allow myself to be entombed in a brace. The lesson I took from this was simple: speak up for yourself.

The Do-Wop Trio

A patient can't really have "evening plans" in the hospital. Something about the hospital gown puts a damper on dating. But John was set to arrive for dinner and a movie — okay, cafeteria food for him, a hospital tray for me, and a show on the TV — at 6 p.m., and I actually fixed up a little. Then it arrived: the gurney, wielded by a small man from "downstairs." It was 5:30, a half hour before my dinner date, and this guy thinks I'm going to levitate off my bed and on to the gurney to be wheeled away.

"No," I said. "Come back tomorrow."

"No?" he asked, incredulous. Patients can't refuse. His eyes darted furtively as if someone might explain, but he was the only one in the room besides me. He wielded his largest weapon, "Doctor wants X-ray today."

I was vanquished but I made no effort to move.

"You have to come here," he indicated the gurney alongside my bed, as if I was going to hop right on it.

"I can't." That much was true, though the fact bought me only a few moments.

He went and came back with the giant lifters, who immediately overpowered me onto the thin mattress, and he whisked me out of my room. By now it was 5:45.

Down the halls, down the elevator, then out into hallways that had no carpeting, I was abducted. Finally I was parked in a dim, mostly empty holding room that reminded me of a scene from the movie "Coma," where bodies lay in a row unattended, waiting who-knows-how-long or for what. It had to be six o'clock by now, so I supposed John had entered my room and discovered I was gone. I'd just taken narcotic pills and it was time for some other meds.

Another "wheeler" appeared and took me into yet another dim industrial room. Giant machines loomed on every wall. This is when the experience tilted. The brisk young women who comprised the X-ray day-shift (I'd met them before) had gone home. This was the night shift. Maybe it was some aberration of the medicine, but I had an image of these three Black men as a do-wop trio from the 1950s. They were harmonizing on a street corner, their heads wrapped in "do rags" (head scarves). I'd fallen into "Little Shop of Horrors" where everything sings. These three — two middle-aged men and one who was younger and good-looking with a meticulously etched hairline (no doubt, the star who was bent on leaving the group for a solo recording deal) — were wearing the regulation blue X-ray uniforms. But as the meds tangled in my system, the image changed and they were wearing tuxedos ... satin ... pastel.

The star motioned to the gray metal object on the wall and asked if I could stand there, offering me his spotlight. At least he had the presence of mind to ask.

Not only couldn't I stand, but I couldn't get out of bed unassisted, and these guys weren't nurses. They conferred in the wings.

The star came back, "Do you want us to help you?"

Remember, I'd missed half my pills and something was really going to hurt soon. It must have been at least ten after six, and up on the eighth floor, I guessed John was asking the nurses where I was. I hoped someone knew and explained. While I was processing all that, the trio lifted me, and pressed me against the cold metal plate. I hung on for dear life to a metal bar over my head.

"This won't take long," the star tried to reassure me.

But after the first picture came another angle and another. In between they checked each plate, while I clung to the bar. At long last, they let me lie down. Now I could see the clock on the wall: 6:30.

"Can I go back now?" I gasped.

They conferred again. I could see them through the glass partition into the next room, no doubt the sound studio where they over-dubbed the chorus.

"He has to make sure the images came out," the star explained.

One of the others had taken all the plates "upstairs" for processing. Up there, someone else had to sign off on them before he could catch the elevator back down. If the shoot wasn't all right, they'd have to repeat the whole thing.

That's when I started negotiating: "Look, I need my pills, I need my dinner, and my husband's looking for me on the eighth floor. How about just letting me go and if the pictures don't work out, take all the time you need tomorrow."

That furtive blink, the same as I'd seen from the gurney man — patients don't make bargains.

I pressed, "If it turns 6:45 and he's not back, I'm out of here, okay?"

Of course, I was bluffing. Exactly how did I suppose I was going to get out of there anyway?

Around 6:45 the bass singer did return ("do do do wop"). They conferred (their final chorus) and for a grand finale I was wheeled away by 7:00.

Upstairs, my dinner had turned cold, but John was waiting in my room watching TV.

And in the corner "Audrey II," the flowering plant from "Little Shop of Horrors," grinned in satisfaction.

May 27

≈

Getting Sprung

I didn't think I was ready. For several days, nurses asked "Going home tomorrow?" and Dr. Pashman had surprised me with, "Well, you want to go home?" That scared me. I was only beginning to hobble to the bathroom and though I was finally able to creep around the corridor leaning on my walker and the rehab person, I couldn't get out of bed by myself, I was still partly bandaged, and I needed a nurse to put me in the shower, dry me off, and lift me back in bed. My IVs had been removed a couple of days before, but instead of the hydrating drip, my primary cuisine was pills, not food. How could I leave the hospital?

And why were they insistent? In truth, hospitals are lousy places to get well. No matter how careful everyone is to be sanitary, the building is full of sick people, and sick people have germs. I didn't contract an infection, but I've heard horrible stories (from other hospitals) of healthy people who went in for a small elective procedure only to contract resistant staph and end up dead. Getting out of there was a good idea. Also, Dr. Pashman mentioned that patients recover more quickly at home, though I didn't see why I'd do better without skilled help.

Another reason occurred to me on May 27. Memorial holiday weekend was coming; doctors didn't want to spoil a three-day vacation to show up and the nursing staff was waiting to flee. Anyone they could get off the floor was one less case, and I noticed a few rooms where people seemed fortuitously "well."

Later, I realized Pashman was right. Psychologically, being home does encourage you to reclaim your life. In my case that worked because my family could help. Still, even the staff wasn't sure. I received momentous "evaluations" from a social worker, doctors, and the rehab department. They convened and presented me with three options — I could be moved to the rehab facility on a different floor within the hospital where I'd have a room but no medical care. Instead, the rehab specialists would work with me for up to three hours each day. This would go on for a week, maybe two. I pictured weeks more in the hospital, in the same hospital gown, being put on and taken off a toilet, walking up and down corridors on a leash.

Or, I could be sent to a convalescent home with 24-hour care outside the hospital if my insurance would pay. That's for people who can't take care of themselves at all. Think nursing home. Think old age home. Think people lying idle in beds for years, rotting away amidst the urine smells of halls tended by underpaid workers.

That's unfair, I know. I'm sure some convalescent facilities are bright and focused on actually convalescing in the sense of getting better. But I thought of the only one I'd ever entered the year voting booths were moved into the "community room" of a nursing home nearby.

While I waited to vote, I was fascinated by their weekly activities board, how hard someone must have worked to find entertainment, or at least a reason to get up in the morning. "Dear Abby" was prominent in prime-time (between breakfast and lunch) every day. A youngish man stepped next to me and asked if I was interested in what they were doing. He was the activities director, it turned out, and he explained with enthusiasm that the staff read "Dear Abby" to the "residents;" it was the height of their morning and they talked about the printed letters for the rest of the day.

I wanted to believe I could theoretically feel okay placing an elderly relative here, partly because he wanted it to be true. But when he gave me a tour, pointing out features like a private television in each room, I'm sorry that all I saw were bodies who looked abandoned, dead eyes watching the flickering screens.

Now, no one was pressing to send me there, at least not exactly. But the possibility was threatening in itself. Was I really that bad? That helpless? That close to dying?

In the light of those possibilities, option three felt like the jail gates swung open: Just go home.

May 27

≈

From Raya's Journal

Last Saturday, my mother left the ICU for a regular room.... Six days later my friends and I buried Linda Martinez.... Tomorrow, mama comes home, home from the cliff's edge, back to our arms.

May 28

~

Going Home

On the morning of Saturday, May 28th, I put on the navy blue knit dress I'd packed two weeks before, and the shoes I'd worn when I'd first walked into the hospital. A nurse helped me into the armchair, and I brushed mascara on my eyelashes. Papers would have to be signed officially releasing me, and before they let me go, the doctor hesitated. Was I absolutely sure someone was at home to help me? Yes! I insisted, anxious to be sprung.

I ate breakfast — it was almost lunchtime — the nurse brought my regular pills as if I wasn't really getting out; and then, there was no one. Wasn't anyone coming for me? Then John and Raya walked in, smiling. I stood up bravely holding the walker and marched to the door by myself. Yes, I'd survived and I was going home.

After

June 1

≈

Home

Five days home from the hospital, I've developed a routine — a series of rituals that divide the day or mark the passages of hours, which don't quite make up days, but are really segments between the pain pills. Not that I'm in so much pain, actually. My left side, where a rib was sawn off, where the team of doctors entered the front of my spine and laid bits of bone between the vertebrae — that hurts — especially between 4:00 and 4:30 every morning; that is, between the 2 a.m. and 6 a.m. pill. But, in all, I'm better every day, and now I'm sitting in the backyard able to write for the first time in two weeks.

My back is held vertical in a straight kitchen chair by the hard white plastic brace surrounding me from chest to torso. I named it *braceosaurus*, as if *brace* was merely a nickname — the thing is too immense for so short a word; it's more like a prehistoric beast the way it holds me in its jaws. Every morning John winds the brace around me stiffly, pulling its Velcro straps to close as tightly as possible, but the monster still overwhelms me. The brace guy measured me right after surgery when I was so swollen my shape scarcely resembled any form I've ever had. Still, he insisted it fit fine. Maybe all hard-shelled *braceosauri* devour their prey like this. In any case, from the start I was told I wouldn't be able to put it on by myself, so the brace became an early evidence of both immobility and dependency.

Not quite *lack of volition* though. After all, here I am, on soft green grass, facing two orange trees — albeit one, which used to bear lush round oranges, suddenly reduced to one last orange the week before I went to the hospital. "It needs vitamins," the gardener diagnosed, as he poured a huge bottle at its roots — though two weeks later it still has only the one orange. I am, on the other hand, taking my vitamins, and despite sitting like a statue, I actually feel full of promise.

Behind the orange tree is an avocado tree abundant with leaves, though it never had a single avocado until this year. We all made remarks about the tree's sexual preferences, though I doubt it was goaded or embarrassed into propagation — more a matter of an improved sprinkler system.

Behind the avocado stands a line of hedges as tall as the trees, which block the prying eyes of the Changs, our neighbors on that side who have finally quit complaining that our branches are in their yard. (Though, at twilight, I did see Mr. Chang's arm surreptitiously reaching through a break in the screen of branches with a saw in hand.)

I am grateful for this serenity. Other spine patients have been in the hospital around three weeks. I was out in twelve days. Some people go home alone, with only visits from a hired helper. I think that would be terribly difficult now that I see the kind of attention involved. And some people, even with loving help, are confined indoors without a mental escape to alleviate their physical entrapments. In a way that I hadn't expected during my busy work-days I appreciate my family and the grass at my feet.

Before surgery, the former patients I'd asked complained of one problem worst of all, worse than pain and their inability to fend for themselves: their children. One man troubled over his two-year-old son who didn't understand why daddy couldn't pick him up and pleaded tearfully every day.

The most egregious cases were older children, eleven and thirteen, who kept demanding that their mother make their lunches, help with homework, wash their laundry, all the services they'd relied on before her operation. The woman could barely walk, and the brats didn't let up whining and complaining. I can interpret this as their way of asserting that nothing had changed, their attempt to cope with fear, denying that they might have lost their mother. But when she confided in me, I couldn't help wondering why she hadn't stood up for herself long before, and why she felt she ought to carry this burden alone.

Now that's a scoliosis metaphor: the spine curves and gives way under the burden of too much weight, not your own, but carrying other people.

As for me, I've been relieved of these pressures by a wonderful daughter in her twenties who keeps trying to feed me, and a husband who in the past had been absorbed in his work in outer space tourism and design, but has grown up within weeks to take responsibility for everything I need.

He helps me out of bed each morning, puts on my brace, helps me into the bathroom, carries my breakfast to the table, puts a pillow at my back, and pushes in my chair. Later, he lifts the "three-in-one chair," which raises the toilet seat a few valuable inches and relocates it to the shower. He takes my brace off again and helps me into the shower. After he steadies me as I step out — so carefully — he dries my back and legs.

"This is the first time I've ever dried a woman coming out of the shower with all my clothes on," he commented sweetly.

This is a mellow time, a gift that has made us a family when in the past we'd often been individuals sharing a house. Yesterday, Phoebe, the cat, killed a bird and deposited it specifically in my office — an offering, I've been told.

So here I sit in a chair on the grass surrounded by artifacts of support. The single most useful tool I brought from the hospital is the "grabber." Insurance covered part of the price; I think it cost around $20. Three feet long of silver metallic plastic, the grabber features a black plastic claw at one end that opens by a trigger and handle at the other. It has a one-inch metal knob to pry open doors and a small magnet on the tip. "FeatherLite" is engraved on the claw. Since I'm unable to bend, this little device has become my buddy. Besides that, I have bottled water, a tissue, this journal and nothing more. After all, what would I do with anything else when I can move so little? Now everything is simplified to its essence.

Patience, healing, a backyard, and a few people who care for me make a surprisingly lovely time.

June 3

≈

Rust

The bills came. Well, so much for the bubble of peace. Insurance on our three cars — mine which waits un-driven, John's and Raya's. Next are cell phone bills, regular phone bills, cable TV (now over $100 each month), my IRS installment with documents and proofs to be signed and sent back, all the utilities, and the first trickle of medical statements.

It's like water beginning to seep from the bottom of a hot water tank. No such thing as a minor problem because that kind of leak signifies rust; it means the bottom of the heater is beginning to fall away, and soon comes the flood.

So here are the first few: some X-rays, three from the anesthesiologist (each for a different amount), one from the main doctor, one from another doctor whose name I don't recognize, two different accounts from the hospital — one of which billed the wrong insurance company, the other asking if I'm insured at all, and two "explanations of benefits" from my insurance carrier, each of which paid at a different incorrect rate. And that's just the start.

The final envelope is from the outside administrator of my disability pay. Now, I've paid into a private disability plan for 23 years — that's my own money that's been amassed by them — and obviously I can't work. You'd think I might get a message reassuring me my disability payments were starting, maybe even wishing me well. But no. The form letter informs me of a "partial denial" while I was in the hospital — as if maybe I was supposed to go to work on a stretcher. That's followed by a "waiting period" of one more week, whose only effect would be to hold back my next monthly pay by 25%. And I don't have the stamina to argue anymore.

Rust at the base of my bubble.

June 6

≈

Three Weeks Ago....

Three weeks ago today at this hour of the mid-morning I was in my first surgery. Faithfully, in the hope of rising above my circumstances, I carried this journal into all the hospital rooms. By writing about the events, I would stand outside them, analytically distanced, coping by placing the pain and details of my care in parcels of words separate from my spirit. Raya and I even joked about the loopy drugged-out prose that would wind all over the page.

But none of that happened. In the early days I was too weak to do anything, asleep most of the time. Then in my four days in the ICU I couldn't have any possessions while they monitored my heart. When I was back in a real room, I did nothing but watch TV — CNN reports over and over interspersed with the "E True Biography" of Jack Nicholson at least twice. I didn't even read the book I'd brought. Exhaustion and resignation were feelings I hadn't anticipated. Only now, when I'm home, can I look back on those twelve days and remember.

June 6

≋

Imagining the Palm Tree

I find I'm too in the moment, too involved with my body to remember anything today. It's been this way despite my higher intention to emerge wiser from the spiritual cleansing of pain, or even just more spaced out from the drugs. Instead, I'm more rooted in physical minutiae than ever.

Years ago, I was in my twenties when I won an Urban Journalism Graduate Fellowship, an honor given by the University of Chicago intended to allow new writers a few months of support while we generated an "important" work — research or even a book. I arrived in Chicago and in the first week fainted and knocked out my front teeth. I never knew if it was a flu, or maybe hunger (I'd been an itinerant artist before winning that nice gig). So instead of writing anything, I spent my fellowship — January to June — in a dentist's office having my mouth re-built.

Unlike my recovery now, that dentist's chair became a kind of lotus pod, or if that's too high-flung, at least it was the portal from which my mind would escape. I needed to avoid the horror of being without front teeth, and later wearing a temporary plastic bridge that belonged in a Halloween costume, and the specter of emerging months later with a face somewhat changed from the person I'd seen all my life, so I powerfully willed myself elsewhere.

Chicago in the winter was relentlessly bitter, even indoors, so I imagined a palm tree, though I'd only seen them in photos. The palm tree stood on a hill in the sunshine with a mountain on one side, the ocean on the other, and I was standing in that light hanging painted cloths (artwork) I'd created. Every day, I pulled my thoughts to that palm tree, to the sunshine.

A few months later, I received a job offer in Los Angeles — here I saw the place I'd so desperately imagined on top of Topanga Canyon.

I'd hoped that after this surgery I'd emerge with a new wonder, a powerful desire that would transform my future like it had decades ago. Instead, I seem to be stuck in an effort to de-toxify my intestines after all the chemical gunk in the hospital. Today I decided to try reducing the painkillers because I don't want any more poison (though I'm glad I have them when I need them!). Sorry to go from sublime to ridiculous but much of my day is spent in the bathroom now.

Not exactly the dream of a palm tree in the sun.

I'll try again tomorrow.

June 9

≈

First Post-Op Doctor Visit

The single image which shadowed the first checkup, about three and a half weeks after surgery, was the woman waiting in the X-ray chairs. Frail and alone, she was breathing hard and shallow. Though I could tell from her expensive haircut that she had, even recently, been amongst the world, maybe even sophisticated or sought at social events, she sat in bedroom slippers, unable, unwilling even, to bother with shoes. Her eyes were half closed but I asked if she'd had spine surgery too. Yes, she breathed, four weeks ago, and the pain has not let up. I asked her where it hurt, and all she managed was "spine."

"Your whole spine?"

"Yes," she whispered.

I asked who her doctor was. Different from mine, it turned out. She was taking Darvocet for pain after the generic of Vicodin stopped working for her. That was all she could say. Yet there I was walking on my own with only a little pain into X-ray.

Why had we fared so differently? One answer may be the doctor's skill. I was lucky. Dr. Pashman, my guy, does "hundreds and hundreds of these," he says; almost two per week, I think. And he has assembled a medical team whom he counts on every time. But who is to say her doctor doesn't do as much? I would advise anyone considering this operation to do some research.

I can't actually take credit for exhaustive checking, partly because my regular doctor, whom I trust, recommended only Dr. Pashman, and, no small consideration, he's the only one my insurance would cover. But I also asked around. I interviewed one of his former patients and asked everyone I knew if they knew anyone who'd gone through this. After a while, the same names came back (spine surgeons are a small community). I'd also had a "second opinion" from a rival institution where the surgeon wouldn't say a word about my doctor but verified that the procedure was necessary. For the frail woman, who's to say more advice would have mattered?

I also took other precautions, and the doctor agrees that the way I went into the surgery made the difference in why I came out "way ahead of the curve" in his estimation, "the bounce-back queen." For six months, I worked on physical training: Pilates one-on-one with a highly-skilled instructor twice a week and I tried to go to the gym for aerobics two more times. On off days I walked. If I could have afforded it, I would have gotten a trainer at the gym too, though prioritizing Pilates turned out wise in strengthening my core so I was walking again soon.

I ate conscientiously always, having been told that intestinal problems are a common post-surgical complaint. Few people could be as careful as I am, but I think any improvement helps. I eat no refined sugar or flour, no wheat, very little dairy, no red meat, no fast food, nothing deep fried, and I take a wealth of supplements. My diet was impossible to follow during the twelve days of hospital food, but I think it let me enter the surgery clean.

And finally, I hadn't been taking any pain medicines. That's not possible, of course, for people who are having the surgery because they're in excruciating pain, but I was fortunate to have had the operation before dire consequences had set in, so afterwards, a smaller amount of pain medicine went further for me.

I was aware that the sad woman might have been me, and whatever the reason I was living, and she wasn't really, my heart went out to her, and I was grateful I wasn't doing as badly.

That said, this post-op visit occurred on the sickest day since I'd been home. The problem wasn't pain, which was tolerable with the pills. The problem was the medicine — Codeine and Tylenol — which made me nauseated, constipated, headachy, unable to eat, and too tired to get out of bed. It was a nasty cycle of being unable to eat and move, which would soothe the medicine, thus making it even more difficult to do anything before I needed another pill for pain. Bad business. I tried getting off the vicious things altogether but it was too soon; my lower back hurt. So, oddly, on this day that the doctor proclaimed me the bounce-back queen, I felt like something that goes in those "caution — toxic waste" or "biohazard" bins.

A simple solution, which worked somewhat, was not to take a pill on an empty stomach. So I put a yogurt (actually soygurt) cup or some dry cereal on my night table, and when I took a pill at 2:00 or 4:00 a.m., I ate a few spoonfuls first. I also cut the pill in half. Instead of a whole dose every six hours or so, I took half a dose with food every four hours.

As Raya and I left, relieved the X-ray looked fine, and all the little bone particles were fusing around the metal rods, integrating them into my body as they should, I was picturing the woman in the X-ray chairs, and by comparison, I knew I'd get past this day.

June 11

≈

A Pain in the Butt

My buns hurt, or glutes, I should say. It isn't funny. Buoyed by
the doctor's release to walk as much as I want, I (foolishly, it
seems) embarked on what, for me, was a major voyage to the
Whole Foods market about seven blocks away. Telling Raya I
might not make it, thereby reserving the possibility of turning
back, I set off using my shopping cart as a walker. I was beyond
my street, comforted that all the houses and trees were as I'd
left them, and achieved the finish line at the store, whereupon I
had to sit down and recharge with a peach smoothie. Somehow
I managed to creep back with our few groceries. But last night
began the revenge of the rear muscles that hadn't worked for
weeks. So I'm taking it easy.

Every day is a new normal: how much I can do, how much is
too much, which pains are for healing (like growing pains), and
which say to respect the process that's still fresh.

Time. I hear the musical adaptation of Ecclesiastes: "There's
a time for every purpose." This time stretches amorphously, lan-
guidly, almost like a summer vacation I never had — if it didn't
hurt so much.

Reality Check

I want to let you know this isn't easy one month after surgery, even though I'm getting along better than most people who've had the same procedure. This isn't to complain, but a reality check for what you might expect several weeks out.

I have six pretty good hours between lunch and early evening, which is when I write this book, so my recovery might sound easier than it is. Although my afternoons are punctuated by naps and pills, I can keep going. But I dread the night — every night.

I know that as soon as the pain pill wears off, at 2:00 or 3:00 or 4:00 in the morning, I will be wakened by a shock that crosses my tailbone and radiates down my legs. Since I've learned that I can't take a pill on an empty stomach, I force myself up on my arms, and then to sit, though I still have a pinch point at my hips that forces a grimace just short of a shriek, as I dangle my legs over the side of the bed. I now keep food near the bed, yogurt or dry cereal, and as much as I want to grab the pill, I make myself eat a few bites first. Then I take the pill with lots of water (also kept by the bed) and struggle to stand. I don't sleep with the brace on, and I can stand without it, but I wonder whether something is pressing on the tender spots.

I lean on the walker parked near my bed to get myself to the bathroom. One effect of the pain pill is to slightly increase urine, which worries me because that might suggest my kidneys are being affected. Still, I have no choice about the pills. By the time I make it back to bed and manage to lift my legs to "log-roll" to lie flat, the pain from my hips down my legs is worse. The pill takes twenty minutes to work, so I lie staring at the clock, waiting for relief. This routine goes on once or twice every night: If I take a pill at 2 a.m., I'm due four hours later at 6:00.

At least as bad as my nights are my early mornings. If I haven't had enough food with the pill, I wake up unable to eat breakfast, feeling sick. Still, I've learned to force myself out of bed because once I get moving and do eat, I gradually feel better. So I push myself up past the pain point and ask John to put on the brace.

If it's a good day, I can manage a bowl of plain oatmeal and coffee (which works better for me than any laxative). The effort of breakfast after a bad night tends to send me back to bed, now in my brace, having eaten. After resting, possibly falling back to sleep for a half hour, I rally to take a shower.

John moves the special chair from its place above the toilet into the shower stall, and helps me step over the ledge and sit under the water. From here on, I begin feeling better. The hot water on my belly relaxes me and I remember how good showers used to feel. Afterwards, John holds me as I guide my feet onto the rubber mat we've placed on the floor, and he dries where I can't reach. Remember, no bending, so my lower legs and feet are distant terrain. Finally, I pull on a simple dress that needs no fastening, and John closes the brace over it.

I don't have energy to stand while fixing up, so I take my cosmetics to sit on the side of the bed. Yes, I believe it's important to dress and put on make-up every day, even if I'm seeing no one. I'm seeing myself, and I need to believe that I'll be okay. Then, dressed and in as good shape as I can muster, I sometimes have to lie down again for another half hour. Meanwhile, I'm counting off four-hour intervals before the next pill.

As I've said, I don't love these drugs — a generic of "Lortab" made of Codeine and 500mg Acetaminophen (Tylenol). Both a nurse and a doctor told me it's safe to take up to 4 grams of

Tylenol a day (4000 mg), so when I was taking a whole pill every four hours, that's 6 pills a day which is 3000 mg of Tylenol. But I wonder if their numbers are based on what's safe for a 200-pound man and asked if it's equally safe for a 110-pound woman. Now I'm taking half-pills, I'm down to 1500 mg of Tylenol a day, and I yearn for the day I can cut back more.

I roll myself to sit, pull up to stand, and I'm ready to try to eat again. If I can, I'll be okay for hours. Throughout the day, Raya and John continue with their appointments and issues, and that takes my attention. I think that if I were living alone, I would dwell on each ache and spasm more. A whimpering mass writhing in self-pity can't get well. So I walk somewhere every day, even if only to the corner mailbox; I resolutely turn on my computer and answer my emails; I talk on the phone; I argue with some of the letters to the editor on the op-ed page of the newspaper; I act like I'm part of the world of the well, though the dread of the next night and morning never quite dissipates.

Patience, I'm learning, is the test here. Recovering from spine surgery doesn't take a few weeks, and the increments of improvement are sometimes small. Fervently, I believe I'll be fine again, and that helps me through these days.

Milestones

I cross tiny milestones every day. Not the leap to freedom yet, not the ability to get in my car, though I understand anew how teenagers feel anxious for their driver's license and a chance to make a two-ton car take them away at their will. That's still a dream, like walking fast or taking big steps or putting my legs on a chair and straightening them, or the great fantasy of getting through a night without pain meds.

I want to focus on little successes: A few days ago, I started leaving the walker in another room and going off on my own legs. My balance is fine, so why not? It's not as if I made a momentous decision (and I still take the walker when I'm outside the house, just in case), but it was as natural an evolvement as a baby's first steps.

The next success was a little surprise. Since I came home, I've entered the house through the yard to avoid the three front stairs. Then, without thinking, John and I started for the local restaurant, and there I was on the steps. One, and the second foot comes with it; step two, then the other foot; stand still for a moment; okay, finally one foot after the other reaches solid ground.

I rode in a car a couple of weeks ago for the brief doctor checkup, strapped into the back seat, surrounded by pillows. But yesterday, I rode for fun, sitting in the front seat "like a person," I told Raya, who was at the wheel. And to think I'd taught her to drive just seven years ago.

We were going to the bank where I expected the security alarm to detect my metal rods and turn me in as a robber. I imagined the SWAT team charging and insisting I turn in my weapons (by ripping them out of my back, perhaps?) or at least holding me in an interrogation cell under a hot light. So we decided Raya would push through the door and alert the guard while I waited outside. I peeked through the glass to watch her talk; he waved me in. With every step, I expected to find out how a bank alarm sounds. But nothing happened. Apparently, the amount of metal isn't enough, he guessed, though that made me wonder what else could get through with just as small an amount of metal. Some day I'll find out about airport alarms.

And finally, this morning I put myself in the shower, stepped out, and dried off by myself. Granted, I still needed help with the brace, but, hey, I did it.

All these little victories are like lights slowly coming back on, one by one, after a blackout, and they measure my days.

June 23

≈

A Terrible Night

Last night was the worst since my days in the hospital. Six weeks out, I'd really hoped I'd be better than this. At 1:00 in the morning, the searing pain that crosses my tailbone to my lower hips and travels down my legs woke me. I raised myself on my elbow to grab for a pill and water and as many bites of a granola bar as I could muster. Then it got worse.

Attempting to stand, I grabbed the handle of my walker that I keep parked next to the bed every night, but when I pulled up, my hips and legs hurt too badly to hold me. Leaning on the walker with all my weight, I made it to the bathroom and back. Rolling into bed hurt even worse.

As I've done too many nights, I watched the clock, waiting the twenty minutes for the pain to subside as I shifted my legs in vain to find any position for relief. This time reprieve didn't come in twenty minutes or thirty. I woke John and asked him to bring ice packs from the freezer. They didn't work much either.

Meanwhile, a raccoon we named George had invaded the kitchen through the cat door and was washing Phoebe's (the cat's) dry food in her water bowl while Phoebe stared, her fur puffed as large as it could get, which was a fraction of George's size. John was out there snapping a towel to drive George out, which apparently wasn't happening either. As I lay in the bed I could hear John trying to reason with the raccoon. It was 2:30 before George left, and John rescued Phoebe, closed the cat door, and returned to bed. I was still awake.

I must have dozed for a while because I woke to the numbers on the clock-radio glowing 4:30. This time I would outwit the pain and not try to get out of bed. I took a pill and lay back down. 5:00. 5:30. At 6:00, I woke John and asked him to put on my brace. I got up. Once I was walking and sat down to breakfast, I felt better. But this can't go on every night.

Around 9:00 I phoned the doctor's office. Of course, he wasn't in. And the next appointment is two weeks away. I settled for that and the assistant's sympathy. It's only been six weeks, you're still healing, he offered, If it's still a problem two months after surgery "we can do some tests, an MRI ... to see what's wrong...."

That part didn't sink in until later: Dear God, not something wrong, not back to the hospital, not the specter of corrective surgery; no more anesthesia and bed pans and hospital gowns; no going back, please!

June 25

≈

Energy

I should have known better. It's just that I wanted so much to be well, to go with a nice couple who are John's friends to dinner and a movie. I really thought I could. It was a Saturday night, soon enough after the Solstice that the sky was still a bright, clear blue at 5 p.m., and a breeze, which promised a soft ocean, wafted over the yard. I ate a bowl of plain oatmeal and downed a half pill, fixed myself as well as I could, put on earrings for the first time since I'd gone to the hospital, and got into the car. Surely, the pill would keep the pain away long enough, and anyway, I'd brought a second half pill for after dinner.

Strolling on the Third Street Promenade in Santa Monica that I've always loved for its crowd and street performers, the Peruvian flute band next to the Michael Jackson imitator, next to the psychic cats and classical pianist, I glimpsed my reflection struggling along clinging to John's arm. There, beside the young woman ambling easily in her jeans and tank top, I looked like an old woman.

Someone at my hair salon had warned me that pain shows on your face. Beyond the muscle mass lost lying in a hospital for two weeks are the etchings on your face left by each pain even after it has passed. Still, I was going to prevail tonight. I managed some conversation at dinner, though as the meal went on, I found myself sinking deeper into the pillow I'd brought from home. Just in case, I popped the second half-pill before entering the movie — so what if it was three instead of four hours after the previous dose.

"Batman" isn't really my kind of film, but John wanted to see it and the couple thought it would be fun. I succeeded in and out of a theater bathroom that didn't have the raised seat I use at home. I made it into the theater chair with barely a wince. Okay, okay now.

But I should have known better. The issue isn't pain. It's energy: the core stamina, the inner strength to heal. I just hadn't understood. By the time I sat in the theater, I had no pain, but I was utterly wiped out. From what? Riding in a car, sight-seeing, and sitting in a restaurant? I guess that's how energy works, more subtle than how much you exercise your body; it's also how much you ask of your mental state.

As the movie blasted on, the second pill kicked in. With all my focus on how much acetaminophen I'd been ingesting, I'd disregarded the codeine, a narcotic. Now it was upon me. I closed my eyes because I couldn't take the assault of images. Instead, every explosion and shout from the screen tore through a narcotic web which interpreted it into a nightmare whose action pillaged what was left of my stamina.

"I wasn't ready yet," I told John later, not wanting to spoil everyone else's evening.

"You did great. The evening worked out very well," he answered.

June 28

≈

The Brace

Elderly Max Lerman, slight and smiling, shook hands with me and my friend who'd driven me to have my brace re-fitted, and all my intentions of complaining drained away. Certainly, I didn't tell Lerman I called the thing a *braceosaurus* or felt devoured by his craft.

When Lerman's rep first came to my hospital room he told me the story: Max had escaped Nazi Germany and fled to China in the 1930s. There, he began making back braces.

Now, I have to stop to form a picture of China in the 1930s, and his devices which must have been wood since plastic hadn't been invented yet; and then I wonder who in that place and time needed a brace or could afford one. The more I plunged into the mystery, the more peculiar the image became.

Nevertheless, I was told that this Jewish youngster in China did so well with his braces that he was able to immigrate to Los Angeles. Here he found a building for sale in the heart of Beverly Hills on Wilshire Boulevard. Twenty thousand dollars was the price in the 1940s, and he balked at it — would a building in Beverly Hills ever be worth such an investment? But he bought it. Six decades later, Max Lerman must be a real estate zillionaire, even if he never makes another brace. But there I was in the same building, watching the wiry man in his unpretentious front office — open Monday through Friday, no appointment needed — with his few assistants and not one piece of Beverly Hills glamour in sight.

I was ushered into a cubicle, as unassuming as the rest of the store. Mr. Lerman, himself, took measurements and went off with my plastic dinosaur. Honestly, I'd hoped to see prostheses — arms, legs, whatever — hanging on hooks or maybe displays of medieval-looking gadgets designed to hold human parts in place. But the oddest object I found was a jar of adhesives whose printed label advertised "for the whole family," presumably for those who want their relatives sticking close.

In a while, Mr. Lerman returned with the brace trimmed so it is lighter and easier to wear, and he strapped it on me, admiring his handiwork. As I left, I was happy to shake his hand. I felt truly glad that after all his journeys he'd come to a place where he felt so satisfied.

July 4

≈

Freedom

Seven weeks exactly since I went into the hospital, and I'm worried. The pain around my tailbone flares every morning when I get out of bed. At night it even invades my dreams. Yesterday, a dream character started to dance, but had to stop, overtaken by pain. Maybe I'd been wiggling around, dancing in bed. Last night I woke a few times: at 4:00, I was ready for a pain pill; at 6:00 I had to stay in bed and cope until I could get up at 7:00, ask John to put on my brace, and then rev up to breakfast and my next scheduled pill at 8:00. After that, like every other day, I'm better once I'm walking around, and by mid-day, I can do almost everything without help.

Last week when I called the doctor about the pain, his "Tech," named Mike, advised a heating pad at night. He thought the issue might be circulation — lying down for a long time might reduce blood flow and somehow cause the pain. Or maybe the heating pad might relax my muscles. Or it's all psychological. Anyway, it worked enough to keep me in bed all night — the heat, combined with my decision not to irritate the places that hurt by getting up.

Part of the scare is that areas in my low back bordering the pain are numb. I don't know if the numbness or the pain will creep, so I phoned my brother Lance, who is a doctor on the east coast, and he comforted me: As long as my motor abilities aren't compromised, don't worry. I'll see Dr. Pashman on Thursday and this time I'll insist on a real response or an MRI or whatever it takes.

Meanwhile, a delicate breeze plays in the sun, this peaceful Fourth of July, far from the troubles in other parts of the world. When fireworks boom tonight, we don't have to wonder if someone is shooting at us; that would be a great blessing for people on much of the Earth. On our patio, John is placing new ceramic tiles textured in shades of terra cotta and warm browns. Raya holds her guitar on a lounge chair singing a soft Brazilian song. Phoebe is chasing white butterflies on the grass, and on this beautiful Fourth of July I want freedom from this freakin' pain!

July 7

≈

Seventh-Week Doctor Visit

The long-anticipated appointment to stop the terrible night and morning pain (or at least complain about it) had arrived, and the results were — herald the trumpets — nothing. The message could be condensed to a shrug, "You'll get over it." Funny thing, writing this a couple of days later, I think they're right.

As I walked into the Institute for Spinal Disorders, where rows of chairs face a wide-screen TV and friendly receptionists offered to validate my parking, it was difficult to keep my momentum gunning for a fix.

As Raya and I waited, we watched CNN's coverage: bomb victims in London holding bloody bodies in blood-spattered hands. How dare I think about my hurting back while those people searched for someone who'd been on a bus or subway now torn to metal shards?

I do realize the logic of making comparisons is flawed: A third grader has a right to be proud of an A on his arithmetic test without being asked if he'd solved one of Einstein's theorems. Your stuff is your stuff; the 1 to 10 pain scale posted in the exam rooms doesn't ask if you hurt more or less than the patient who was in that room before, only how bad it is for you. Nevertheless, events thousands of miles away gave me pause.

By 1:30 in the afternoon, I felt pretty good as the nice man who'd already consoled me on the phone escorted me two floors down to X-rays.

I pressed him: "It's terrible. I wake up from the pain at night, and it's really bad on my right side when I get out of bed."

He nodded, and smiled, "You just had a very big operation."

A little later I repeated the litany of problems to the nurse in the exam room: numb areas, tailbone, right hip. Dutifully, she wrote everything on the chart before sighing, "I've heard that from two other patients this morning."

Grabbing her forefinger, she illustrated: "If your finger was in a vise for a long time and you took it out of the vise, it would feel good at first. But as the nerves came back it would start to throb." Spine patients commonly have new pain or a return of old pain weeks after surgery. "People are always calling and saying the operation failed, but that's not true."

She scurried away the instant the doctor and his student-doctor entered. Today, sporting a navy pin-striped jacket instead of the usual white lab coat, Dr. Pashman exulted, "The X-rays look great!" He knew I'd called, and raised his eyebrows as I went down the list: ouch, numb, ouch.

He asked about my pain pills and I thought, hey, I'm not trying to knock myself out. I want the pain actually gone. He pointed out that people develop a tolerance to the medication, so since I'd reduced the dose (by cutting the pills in half), in effect I'm taking even less. If he was implying I should drug myself through this, that wasn't the answer I'd come to find.

I ramped up my energy, standing and pointing exactly where I was attacked each morning when I got out of bed, calling it excruciating.

He answered, "Yeah, that happens to me too."

Ummmm, "But you didn't have the surgery."

No answer.

I asked what he did for his pain, and he suggested putting a board under the mattress or trying one of those hot patches that are advertised.

Since I wasn't getting much of a rise, I went for shock value, taking off my brace and drawing the numb areas around the incision sites.

"We had to cut through nerves. Some of them may come back," he commented, unfazed.

And the swelling?

"The band of your pants is making a line," he noticed.

Well, yeah, when you have edema and you press in, it leaves an indentation. But the cause of my back pain wasn't my pants!

I turned to Raya for reinforcement, "Did I forget anything?"

"I guess not," was all she said.

I'd reached the end of show-and-tell without ringing any bells.

Pashman turned to the doctor-fellow and complimented me as "the kind of patient you want. She chose to do this months before and prepared for it. She ate conscientiously; wasn't on any pain medications; she asked good questions; she's intelligent; her expectations were realistic; and she's done great."

Aw, shucks, what could I say after that?

He said, if I still have concerns in a month he can do a CT scan or other tests. "But there's an old saying, if you take a temperature, you'll find a fever. You're right on course."

Leaving, I thought of a character from a decades-old musical, "The Wiz." The show featured a witch who belted out, "Don't bring me no bad news today! Don't bring me no bad news today!!"

Truth is, Dr. Pashman has been through this more than a thousand times. So, okay, I'll trust him — at least until my visit next month.

July

≈

The Fellowship Of The Brace

Jennifer

As I stepped onto the outdoor patio of the Rose Café, I saw Jennifer before me at a small round white table wearing a brace exactly like mine. I stood transfixed while my friend Cathy went to our table. I'd named Cathy "executress" of my will in the dark days of worry before my surgery. Now sunlight filtered through the white gauze above the café, but all I noticed was Jennifer, tall, blonde, in her twenties, none of which describes me; still, I recognized her as a member of my clan. I went to her.

She reacted wide-eyed and pointed at my brace. Like long-lost sisters we laughed in recognition as the identifiers tumbled out: Back surgery? Yes. With the rods? Yes. Where? Cedars, too? Who? Dr. Pashman? You're kidding. He's my doctor!

Inevitably the question common to all members of my clan is spoken: "How many degrees?"

Not quite like comparing S.A.T. scores, but somehow a competitive edge goes to the worst scoliosis curve. My first brush with one-upping came from a former patient I interviewed on the phone before my surgery. My curve was sixty-eight degrees, I told him.

"Gotcha! Mine was seventy-two," he bragged.

Jennifer's was fifty degrees, so I told her it's a good thing she had the operation now because it would have gotten worse.

Actually, in my twenties, my curve was around forty degrees, where it remained for at least a decade before a progressive degeneration of more than twenty degrees over the next decades.

Her surgery was done three and a half weeks ago (a month after mine), yet here she sat looking pretty, able to enjoy her brunch. It occurred to me that she might feel worse before she fully recovered; I'd learned that often some pain kicks back before it dissipates for good, but I didn't want to spoil her afternoon.

We bonded over bad nights and pain in the early mornings, wanting to wean ourselves off the same pain pills, and how she missed touching her feet. Eventually, I left her and went to join Cathy at lunch.

But later when Jennifer waved good-bye, walking out of the café holding her boyfriend's arm, gingerly taking each small step, I watched knowingly and with affection.

DeLane

A man rushed into Marie Callender's from the parking lot, shouting "DeLane! DeLane!" towards the front of the line, pointing at me as I stood just inside the doorway. It was so urgent he edged through the line to a statuesque woman in jeans with short blond hair. She was intent on getting her table, but whatever the man said made her give up her place and come to the back of the line.

I guessed by now: it was the brace, and the greeting was what I was coming to expect: "I wore one just like that."

As with Jennifer, the identifications tumbled out: steel rods, Cedars, Pashman. The difference was time; DeLane was ten months past surgery and confident. She pulled up her shirt and revealed a side scar identical to mine. So they'd done both front and back on her too, probably took the same rib and operated two days apart. We knew secrets about each other — our rites of passage in the hospital.

How many Pashman graduates are around? I fleetingly pictured a drill team — hey, maybe a whole battalion — of good-looking women called, "The Pashettes," showing off their side scars and marching with straight backs, beating drums and blowing those little blue inhalers they gave us in the hospital to inflate our lungs.

Since DeLane was Dr. Pashman's most experienced patient I'd met, I seized the chance to glimpse my own future. How did she feel now?

She planted her feet in a solid stance and proclaimed, "Look, I'm standing in the middle of my legs!"

I couldn't picture her otherwise; she was so comfortable in her body.

"He's the best doctor in the country," she confided, as if I ought to be wise to that too.

I didn't ask if she'd surveyed the whole country. What mattered was that she was so clearly, honestly glad she'd had the surgery.

"Ask me anything," she encouraged me.

I understood how she felt, wanting to share the experience (Hey, I'm writing this book.). But I didn't know where to start, so I asked how soon after her operation she'd started driving. "Several months," was all she remembered, but commented that she was always careful. "Respectful" was her word; respectful of what had been done, of the rods.

What I really wanted to know was how soon all the pain would be gone; when would I be completely all right? In ten months was it finally over? She weighed her answer.

"Pain ... Pain is a personal thing. No, I wouldn't say pain exactly...."

Her table was ready.

The man was already going with the hostess.

"Call me," she offered, handing me her business card.

Maybe I should have, at least to learn the end of her sentence. But I think I know.

Jose

I'd seen him for years at the photo shop, though our conversation had been limited to "double prints, glossy, no borders." I'd never even known his name. If I'd thought about it, I'd have guessed he was forty-ish, probably athletic, maybe meets women at a gym. But today when I walked in wearing a brace, everything changed.

"I wore one like that for six months. It was terrible."

His story began in the early 1970s, and though it gave me no more insight than reading about medieval torture, it did suggest how far spine surgery has evolved. He had three back surgeries, each at small hospitals named for different patron saints that apparently watched over broken arms and the flu but were out of their depth with spines. In fact, I vaguely recalled one of the three being mentioned under a newspaper headline like "State Investigates Missing Patients."

But at nineteen, I guess he had no choice, so in disabling pain, he delivered himself up to a surgeon who removed three discs and inserted "Harrington rods" along his spine. No longer used, these rods had hooks at the top and bottom that grabbed the vertebrae so a surgeon could twist the spine into position. Once there, the spine was wound tightly by wires that risked pressing on nerves.

One effect was that he spun around a central axis, he said. That is, if his feet were forward, his shoulders might be ninety degrees to the left. He showed me how he would reach up and pull a shoulder around, only to have it swing all the way to ninety degrees in the opposite direction. He didn't think it was funny at the time. And everything hurt. On top of that, he was told the rods would break if he ever bent over. So he had the rods removed in a second operation a year later.

Twenty years later, in 1993, he finally had a surgery that worked for him, stabilizing his discs, though this one was a nightmare too. The third hospital placed him in the plastic brace while he was still on the operating table. Within days, he developed blisters from it rubbing against bare skin, and he lived with that for six months.

No reputable doctor or hospital does any of those procedures anymore.

Remarkably, he was glad he'd gone through it anyway. He stands straight, and though he can't lift anything (and doesn't even try going to a gym), he's grateful.

"I would have been in a wheelchair by now."

So after all these years I know his name, Jose, a new friend.

Joyce

I wasn't actually shopping in the furniture section of a department store, just sitting on the furniture, when a woman in her sixties appeared with a broad smile. Joyce wore an elastic support band around her waist and carried an elegant bronze-handled cane.

She began, "I recognized that brace!"

She had a message for me.

I listened avidly for a story from our Fellowship. She said rods like mine weren't in use twenty years ago when she had her first scoliosis surgery at age forty, so her doctor at UCLA implanted another kind.

Joyce was never comfortable with them, but "Nothing ever stopped me," she emphasized. "You learn how to deal with things."

Ten years later she had a second surgery to repair some problem with discs, and had the rods removed. Also, she didn't want the pain medicine in her system, so she went through her recovery "cold turkey" with a nurse packing her in ice until the pain finally subsided.

"Please don't misunderstand," she added quickly, she wasn't relaying all this to scare me, quite the opposite: After that second surgery, she flew to a distant mountain reachable only by helicopter and she hiked to the top.

I looked at her elastic support and the cane, and wondered how well she really was and how much was bravado. Oh, she'd considered having a third surgery, she explained, but she didn't want to go through that anymore, and, anyway, her doctor had died. Many people she used to know had died, but she's one of the most active people in her circle.

"You learn which side of the street to walk on, which part slopes right or left; you learn what works for you; you catch on."

Yet she had the cane.

"This?" she laughed it off, posing on one leg, the other leg crossed at the ankle in a dancing position, one arm on her hip. "As long as I keep moving I'm fine. But if I have to stand still, I just do this."

I asked her if the pain had continued; does it finally go away? Quietly, she admitted it never leaves completely.

"They opened up your body. When the inside of the body is exposed, even just to the air, you have to expect some effects, maybe kind of like arthritis."

She saw I was worried. I'd always hoped I'd be better one day, really all better, back to the way I was before.

Quickly, she touched my arm, and whispered with urgency, "What I want to tell you is it's all right."

Still, I felt sad after she left. I knew she'd meant to encourage me by saying she'd climbed a mountain after her surgery. Yes, I heard that. But I also heard her warn that I'm in a new body now; that I can't go home again, and it's time to make peace with a different kind of future.

July 22

≈

Driving

So, suddenly you find yourself in someone else's body. The comfortable chair doesn't fit anymore; you reach for the familiar handle to open a drawer but it's no longer at your fingertips. You rush to the mirror expecting the image you knew, but instead someone else, perhaps a relative with different proportions, a different balance, looks back at you with puzzled eyes.

From Kafka's, *Metamorphosis,* where Gregor woke up as a cockroach, to all the movies in which a woman is incarnated into a man's body (or the other way around), or a child wakes up as an adult, body-shifting has been a staple of fantasy story-telling.

Except that you don't really expect it to happen to you. Oh, sure, I was warned that I'd be taller and stand straighter. I did notice the cabinet over the bathroom sink was easier to reach. And of course I'd peeked under the brace to notice that my waist had lengthened, happily, and looked more like when I was a teenager. So this didn't seem like an absolute case of body snatchers.

That is until the first time I sat in the driver's seat of the old blue car I'd driven for ten years.

Now, a driver's seat is personal. Those profligate rental cars always feel temporary, reluctant to hug you lest they might become too attached. Through the years, I'd adapted my car to every curve: the seat forward to a precise notch and tilted just so, the small oval white pillow rested perfectly at my lower back (partly to hold up my descending spine), the mirrors at eye level. I trusted all that...

... Until yesterday. The doctor had said I could drive as soon as I felt ready. In fact, he'd given me permission weeks ago. But I just couldn't. What if I twisted my back getting in? What if my muscles began to hurt or spasm in that bad spot near my hip? What if there was too much pressure on an injured nerve or my tailbone, or my reactions were too slow because of the pain pills, or my strength wasn't enough, or, worst of all, what if someone hit my car and I was all alone and the rods in my back broke and they stabbed my lungs and I was lying bleeding in the street and the paramedics were late and then they took me to a different hospital where they had no idea about my surgery ... What if?

But honestly, I can't keep asking John or Raya to drive me on every little errand. And it's nobody else's business if I want to waste a little money while I'm out. Time to be independent. As I approached the first time driving since the operation, I felt like a kid in one of those "Caution — Student Driver" cars. The plan was for John to sit next to me as I'd practice going just around the block and only once. It sounded safe enough.

But from the moment I occupied the driver's seat, everything was wrong. My trusted little white pillow was smashing my brace against my back. Without it, I didn't know how close to sit to the pedals. And the mirrors no longer greeted my eyes. I was different, not just a little taller and straighter; I was shaped like someone else, and my old car no longer knew me. Once around the block, uncomfortable, was all I could stand.

That was yesterday. This morning I set out with an armful of pillows in various sizes and tried each one behind me (little white oval relegated to the back seat, a souvenir). I put another pillow under my legs. My fingers grappled for the levers that move the seat.

And then I went, not just around the block, but far, far away (okay, fifteen minutes away) to the post office. And then I drove home. It was done.

I had inhabited this strange new body a little more today.

July 27

≈

Painting Again

Honestly, I was scared. Chicken. Cowardly. I wasn't sure I'd be able to paint again. Oddly, I never had the same doubts that I'd be able to write after the operation. Unless I had brain damage (which I didn't expect), I was sure I'd be able to finish this book as soon as I had the stamina. Even during the worst times in the ICU, though my heart faltered, my brain never did.

But painting? For me, that seems to come from a different source, less to do with a functioning intellect, psychological insights, or skill with language — it's more a question of whether the pathways to the unconscious, to the Source, are free. It's a delicate link, unpredictable each time, more like a microwave that has energy but no substance and can be stopped simply by interrupting the beam. An operation on my central nervous system, lying unconscious for a total of sixteen hours, concentrating exclusively on my physical survival, and being plied with numbing drugs — now those sound like woolly mammoths positioned between me and any "source."

I already had a precedent for doubt: In the two weeks before I went to the hospital, nothing I painted worked, and the results of being so disconnected are two panels — one with the image blanked out in white; the other went all the way to black spray paint to obliterate my failure. I told myself this was just a pre-op distraction; let this phase pass and everything would come back.

Or would it? I put off finding out. First, painting is a physical activity, especially the way I work. I prefer large wooden "canvases" flat on a table, or spread between carpenter's horses, or lying on the grass. Painting on those horizontal surfaces requires bending, reaching, or even crawling on the ground. We're not talking little pictures placed daintily on an easel where a painter sits, moving only a wrist. That's just not me. So there was a credible excuse — I couldn't go back to painting because I literally wouldn't be able.

John started getting on my case just weeks after I came home: "Why don't you try something small enough to prop in front of you, even while you're in bed?"

After two more weeks doing nothing, his suggestions escalated: "I think it would be good for you if you painted something, doesn't matter what it is; you'll feel better."

I kept watching television. I'd even do the laundry, the dishes. No painting.

A week later, John tried again, "Look, I'll move the things outside for you and set you up. I know how you are — that's the way you'll get well. How about today?"

Grrr, nobody tells me what to do, especially not about art. Emails needed answering.

Then yesterday, finally, the veil lifted. I don't know why. Maybe it coincided with reducing the pain pills, maybe because I was healing, or maybe the energy that originally called me to make art as a teenager finally trickled through the smog of hospital chemicals and weighty events. Whatever — I went into the half of our kitchen we'd fitted out as my studio.

I looked at the all-white painting and the one I'd spray-painted black in frustration. No, I wasn't going to rescue them. This is a new time. I had to be new again the way every artist anywhere is new at the moment of creating any form of art.

And now my first post-op work glows in shades of yellows and gold, colors I hadn't used much before. I was surprised. What finally came from all of this, after all the tribulations, turned out to be full of hope.

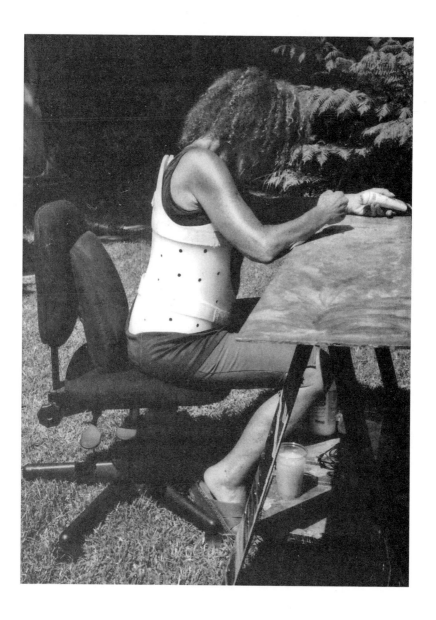

August 11

≈

Third-Month Checkup

Almost three months after surgery I drove myself to the doctor's office. For the first time since the operation, I saw Dr. Pashman without my daughter at my side.

I felt good. I'd reduced the pain pills down to two halves each day — one-half before sleeping, one-half the next afternoon, and they don't upset my stomach anymore. My appetite has returned. The pain in my right hip is gone, I walk faster with larger steps, and I've packed away the metal walkers. The commode/shower chair is finally going to charity; I've rediscovered the joys of sitting on a real toilet and standing in the shower.

Of course, I'm still healing, the nurse reminded me, "Even though you feel well, your back isn't well."

Not yet. I shouldn't lift anything, turn, twist, or "fold, spindle or mutilate" (as instructions used to warn on punch-cards). And the bottom of my tailbone still aches sometimes.

The new Spine Institute Fellow (yet another surgeon in training) nodded his head, "That's the coccyx," and he pointed to the tail at the bottom of the plastic spine in the exam room. "It gets inflamed. No one knows why. Try sitting on one of those donut cushions."

I nodded, privately dismissing the image of carrying a butt pillow with a hole in the middle into a classroom when I return to teaching.

I still have other issues: after months without stretching, massage, or any exercise besides walking, I've lost muscle mass and

I'm stiff. I can't sit cross-legged on the floor anymore because my left leg won't come around. In fact, I've discovered anomalies about my left side which lead me to the heart of this visit....

Little girls in the waiting room: One child, maybe ten, was encased from her armpits to her thighs in a white plastic brace like the one I wore. She carried a pink pillow made of huggable plush held to her pink t-shirt. I knew her mother would have had to tie the pink laces on her white sneakers because the girl couldn't bend. Sleepless nights shadowing her face, the mother led her child with one hand as her other arm grasped a bed pillow. A second woman followed, maybe an aunt, also bearing a pillow and a stuffed creature of indeterminate species, whatever comes in pink.

Everyone else sat watching CNN on the giant screen — I was stuck in the reception area for more than an hour, by myself — but the child's mother pleaded, "She has to lie down right away," and their posse was let in.

A second child entered warily — her first visit, I guessed. She was shaped like a question mark, her belly swayed round in front, her rear slanted back. Probably only nine years old, she trailed a woman who cradled a ringing cell phone and moved like a starlet in high heels. I peered into the child's deep brown eyes and recognized her fear before she turned her gaze away.

I shifted in my chair, couldn't get the pressure off my tailbone, and finally stood. Better. I could feel the new heel lift in my shoe. For a week I'd been raising my left leg with layers of drugstore heel inserts. Everyone is a little different on each side, but it took three-quarters of an inch of foam pads for my shoulders to appear level in the mirror.

Later, in the examining room, I took off my shoes, allowing my left shoulder to drop to demonstrate how uneven I'd become. That's a back surgeon's nightmare. Dr. Pashman's face actually blanched. Quickly, I assured him it wasn't his fault. Still, he defended himself that they'd measured carefully from my pelvis to my shoulders and I was perfectly straight. That's right, I agreed. But my left leg is shorter. Apparently, over the years, my spine had degenerated in a way that collapsed my longer side, which ironically made me stand straighter at forty-five than I had at twenty-five. All these years I'd forgotten that I used to troop to a shoemaker to glue more rubber on the heels of my left shoes. Funny, how you edit away those memories. So, no, my unbalanced sides have nothing to do with the surgery...

... Except that this whole experience brought me back to my childhood, to when I might have had the eyes of the question-mark child. I suddenly remembered one day at a shoe store when I was the age of those children in the waiting room today. Tension pervaded that day, I recall vaguely, probably because the shoes might cost more than my father had. As I tried on a shiny pair of Mary-Jane's, the salesman noticed a slight differ-ence in my walk. At first my dad was offended — he was always on guard against any slight.

Then he weighed the idea, and asked himself aloud, "I wonder if you might have had a touch of polio."

He squeezed my right and left calves and found them equally strong. I always had good muscles.

"No, she's perfect," he informed the salesman and ended the matter.

But now I wonder. When I was a tiny child growing up in New York in the mid-1950s, the City had waves of polio scares, closing all public swimming pools, frightening people with news photos of children in "iron lungs" (immobilized in metal breath-ing machines shaped like barrels), or paralyzed for life without warning. The frenzy had started with President Roosevelt long before I was born. But not until later in the '50s was the vaccine widely given.

One year when I was too young to understand, my brother and I were told we couldn't go outdoors to play all summer long. In New York's heat and with no air conditioning, our windows were sealed shut as we hid from the invisible attacker until the weather turned too cold for the germ, they believed. Thus we survived, all healthy, or so we supposed.

But what if I did have what my father had whispered: "... a touch of polio?" What if the curved spine and the slightly shorter leg went together? No one knows what causes scoliosis. "Genetics" is the usual non-answer, and a disease so clearly structural and mechanical seems far from the iconography of infections — but, what if?

Not that it matters anymore. Those children in the waiting room were probably born with spinal deformities, and I expect their parents had been advised to wait until they'd grown enough for surgery. As for whatever archaic horrors might have been done to my spine in the 1960s, thank goodness for my family's denial that anything was needed. Today's kids are luckier.

I felt lucky on this day too. Dr. Pashman told me my X-ray looked great. I answered that I felt great. I'd graduated. I could take off the brace whenever I want, "it's done," he said (though I still rely on the brace's security, especially in a car).

And for the first time, three months after my surgery, I didn't bring a list of questions, at least none he could answer...

... like why did it all happen? And when will I dance?

Fourth-Month Checkup

Why was I bothering to go back to the doctor when I felt so well I could almost forget I had the surgery? Almost. Never entirely. I'd been completely off pain meds and out of the brace for nearly a month. Sure, it was still awkward to get in and out of cars, and every once in a while I felt a twinge — not quite a pain — in my lower back, maybe one more bit of bone settling into place, adjusting. The rubber tire poking out my abdomen still hadn't yielded to working those muscles in Pilates. But it will. And one day all the pings along my spine will have healed. Not today, but still, why go?

Dr. Pashman put his finger at the middle of my back on my spine and said that's what I had to protect, the place where metal met the bone, where they had to fuse, where I had yet to heal. The X-rays showed I was coming along, but in the darkness under my skin, the bones still needed to grow together, nerves and muscles to entwine the steel, accepting them until metal and flesh were inseparable. That takes a year. Be careful — it could still fail.

But I knew that. So what was the real meaning to take from this last regular visit? After this, I wouldn't return for three months, and then a year, and then never again, assuming all goes well. Strange, in a way. This experience had become so much a part of my plans, even my identity for awhile, that it felt like one of my moorings was coming loose.

When I first came to this office, my book about writing television drama had just been accepted by a publisher. On that day I had looked at the frightening X-ray of my spine and Dr. Pashman told me I really must go through all this. Now, on this day, almost a year later, when I tried to leave my house, the door was blocked by a box. It held advance copies of the published book. So this was a circle.

As I left the Spine Institute near Cedars-Sinai, I was in a hurry to get back to work on a painting, and I had to answer an email from school about my classes when I return next term, and deal with that box of books, and pick up something for dinner and.... All the things that had been interrupted were there waiting for me.

Six months after my first entry in this book, I've come home from the adventure, not the same (no one is the same after a life-threatening, life-saving experience), but I've returned to tell you the story.

Afterword from John

≈

I'm thankful we could get this operation done and fix Pam. I've been very frustrated for a long time because her back condition was getting worse and there was nothing I could do about it.

I'll never forget the day of the operation. We had to get Pam up at 4:30. We'd been all prepared, and everything was packed. We got cleaned up and drove her over to the hospital. There was no traffic. We were waiting for a while, and then the people came out and took her. I remember seeing her walk into the hallway with a few other people and I thought to myself: I sure hope this works out because it is a very serious operation and this could be the last time we ever see her. This is real.

Then, a number of hours later, as you usually see in movies and TV shows, the doctor came out. That happened a few times to other people while we were sitting there; the doctors told them everything was fine. But not us. Instead we got a phone call. I felt like there was this loud music in the background — "dum de dum dum."

I remember counting the paces. I'm an architectural designer so I tend to measure things. It was thirty paces from where I was sitting to the telephone, and half the room was looking at me. I had developed some strategies. If the worst of the worst happened and the doctor came out and said Pam didn't make it, I'd actually planned what I was going to do. I was going to find a chair and just sit there. And the next thing would be to call her brother, Lance. I didn't have a plan after that, but that's what I figured I was going to do. Pam had given me an envelope which I put in my fire safe — "If I croak, here's what you guys should do." That was the right thing. We really approached this in the most calm, organized, almost professional way.

When I picked up the phone, it was Dr. Pashman saying they were all happy. This perpetuates my feeling that we have a sort of lucky star looking over us. There are hard times, frustrations, and constant work, constant work, constant work. But in all we have been very lucky, and I recognize that. I also feel we've been given a gift, so let's make the best use of that gift. Let's really make the household work even better; let's stay cool; let's create stuff.

It all comes to this: understanding what's going on, feeling great that you can have a complex, difficult operation like this, and that medical science is at a point that we can have something like that done. The consequence of not having it is that she would have simply deteriorated. She has a second life. She got fixed. It's absolutely amazing.

Epilogue
Five Years Later

July 2010

≈

Five years later I am well. I have no pain, but I'm aware every moment that I am changed. I don't mean because I have steel rods and screws in my back. So what if I hesitate any time something falls on the floor, having to plan a strategy to pick it up? And if people have to wait for me to get in or out of a car, so be it. None of that matters.

But when I see an elderly person bent deeply over a cane, breathing hard as she struggles down the street, her back in a perpetual "n" for no, my heart goes out to her, not in pity, but in empathy. I sometimes imagine her as a child running with other children, and see that child living in her. I take a moment to send her love, and I want to believe she has joys. A life of pain like that is palpable to me. But it will never be me, not anymore.

In the first months after the surgery — the period encompassed by this book — I was focused on my physical state. Recovery meant returning to all the things I used to do, insisting I wasn't changed in any important way, merely inconvenienced. I'd been a scrappy kid, growing up in New York City, fighting for every job as if survival depended on it, and in some ways it did in those early years. If I didn't die, I intended to get back onto the success track.

I didn't die, but gradually over the next years, I realized that in some ways the person I had been was no longer there. I lived in the same house with the same people and went back to the same job, but I felt like a ghost from the afterlife playing at being me, unwilling to let go of those moorings. It took years — not the healing; I was walking around within months — but slowly it dawned on me that the person who went into that hospital is not quite the one who came out.

The awakening began with gratitude. To this day, every time — every *single* time — I get up from a chair and walk across the room, I am awed by how wonderful that is. Being able to get out of bed and get some water — what a remarkable act. From those small bubbles of light began a larger realization.

I had what I called "vanilla sky" moments, from the movie in which Tom Cruise played a disfigured man in a coma whose "lucid dreams" gave him an alternate reality. All this time was extra, a gift of grace. Had I died in the ICU and all this was a dream? Was I still in a coma, only imagining I had a second chance?

Or did I really have a second chance? As a teenager and young adult I was an artist. I would lose myself in a painting for days while the world went by. But artists don't make money, and the practical survivor in me put away what I loved, all the canvases and brushes, all the colors, all that life for good jobs as a writer. Twenty years went by as I built a career and raised a child. Twenty years.

Actually, I had started to paint again the year before the surgery, so I had already begun reaching back for the person I used to be. But I was still out pitching projects, competing for assignments, negotiating with executives and lawyers, making hard deadlines, working as a university professor, and finishing the glossary on a book.

Then it all stopped. During the worst days — months after surgery when I was able to move around — I took refuge in painting. I would focus on each nuance of color and turn of the brush until the hurt faded beneath the force of the image that was forming — persevering, even when I was barely able to lift the panels on which I painted.

People sometimes speak of "the gift" of an illness, and I wouldn't have understood until it happened to me. I think the "gift" is being forced to ask why you are living, who you truly are. For me, the answer was emphatic: Return to my core as an artist in order to stay alive. You might say that spiritually I was pushed back into what I'm supposed to do in this world.

From my new center, I learned three lessons I want to pass on to you: First, I learned to let go. I took my hands off the steering wheels of my business, my household, my project deadlines, all the *things* that once seemed necessary. I just let go. And, you know what? Nothing crashed. Other people did some of them, and some were undone. Most of it doesn't really matter.

Second, I learned to trust other people. I truly wasn't sure whether my own family could overcome their individual needs to help me. But they grew, and they did it. And so did some strangers.

Third, I learned: do what you care about. This time, this moment is yours, right now.

Astronauts who saw the Earth from outer space speak of "the overview effect," the vision of the Earth as a whole from the perspective of great distance. Picture Earthrise as seen from the Moon. Those images may teach us, not that we are small, but that we are as large as the cosmos we can imagine.

In that spirit, the perspective from this journey through back surgery gave me unexpected peace. Stillness, a *quiet*, came over me once I recovered. I realized one day that after fighting so hard and so long with all the bits and pieces of day-to-day existence, the noise had stopped. It simply stopped.

A yoga teacher once told my class "death begins in the spine" because when you are no longer flexible you can break. Having a spine made rigid was against all I had learned. And yet, somehow, the energy continues to move along that steel path. The nerves have grown around the rods the way the roots of trees twine and reclaim objects deep in the ground. And, in time, the things made by man and the things of nature become one within a universe of endless possibility.

Appendix I

Some Practical Advice

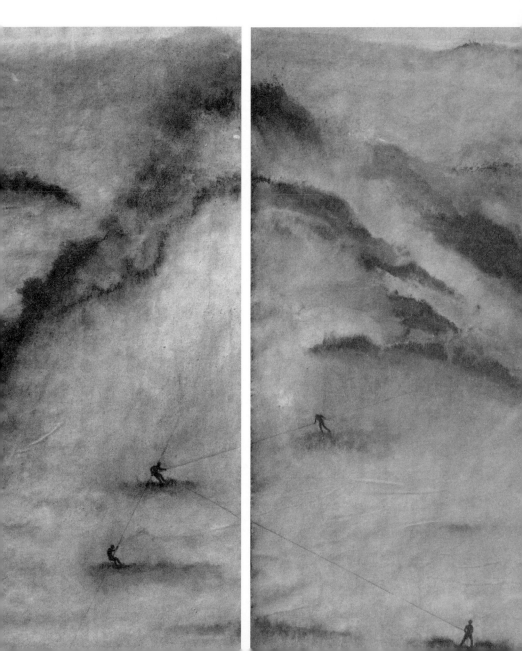

Clothing

Consider two realities after back surgery: You can't bend, and you're wearing a brace. So kiss your feet goodbye before you enter the hospital because you're probably not going to touch them again for quite a while. And, the brace covers any fastenings, including a waist-band, so unless you're able to loosen the brace and re-fasten it throughout the day, the simplest clothes are most practical.

Before surgery, I stored my favorite buckled platform sandals in the closet along with anything on heels and my sneakers that tie. I shopped for flat slip-ons with no laces, buckles, snaps, Velcro, or anything else that might need hands. Once I was up and walking, and my back was sensitive to each jarring step, I liked my soft foam-soled shoes best. Some people recommend bare feet for balance, but I found that shoes gave me more stability.

The medical-supply salesman who visited the hospital showed me a device to put on socks. It looks like a pliable plastic funnel with stirrups. You place the sock over the funnel and lower it to your feet, holding the straps. Slip your foot into the plastic casing and pull up. *Voila!* The salesman omitted how you get the socks off though — prehensile toes, I imagine. And don't try it with stockings; the plastic will snag them to shreds. Personally, I opt out of socks, tights, pantyhose and their ilk until I can sit in lotus position.

I don't know how men manage their long pants. I guess they figure out how to lift their feet into the pant legs, but it's a trick to get that second leg into the tunnel without losing the territory the first has gained or watching the pants pool out of reach on the floor. I guess they could use the grabber to pull the pants up. Once there, closing the waist isn't a problem if they don't have a brace on. But after the brace covers the waist, the only hope of getting those pants down again is to loosen or even remove the brace. That's okay if you have double-jointed elbows or the dexterity and stamina to re-fasten it behind your back. Otherwise, people in pants are likely to need help getting re-dressed. I know because I tried to put on my stretch exercise pants, which I used to wear almost every day. After six weeks, I was able to get my feet in the bottoms while sitting, then reach down and pull. After almost eight weeks, I could put the brace back on by myself after a struggle, but I had the option of wearing a skirt.

In fact, my most useful garment early on, which I wore home from the hospital, is a plain knit dress with short sleeves that has room for a swollen abdomen and hangs straight. I never liked that dress, but under the brace you can't see what it looks like anyway.

Just be sure you have something next to your skin everywhere the brace touches to avoid irritation. You'll sweat under the brace, so you need enough easy-on clothes to last between washes.

For the cold, I relied on ponchos — they slip easily over everything without looking odd, and they hide the brace (if you care to do that). I couldn't button any of my winter coats over the brace, though.

I spoke to one man who wore his brace on top of suit jackets; he once put it over a tux, he said. Not my taste, but who knows, maybe "le brace" will become a fashion statement. Meanwhile, twelve weeks is the minimum for wearing the stylish plastic accessory, and by six weeks I was sporting it everywhere. I didn't care who stared anymore.

Hair

If your hair is boy-cut short, so straight it never tangles, or if you're bald go ahead and skip this little tip. But if you're fluffy like me, in the spirit of "I wish I'd thought about that...," I suggest you do better than I did.

A week before surgery, I went to the hairdresser for everything I'd need to hold me over for a couple of months, which could also be seen as part of my preparation for the prom. The day before I left for the hospital, I washed my hair sparkling clean. None of that lasted.

The problem isn't only that you won't be able to get to a shower to wash your hair while you're in the hospital for a couple of weeks. Nor is your lack of energy to brush your hair the culprit. Sweat is the demon. Picture it (or don't — if you don't want to be grossed out): Lying on a pillow in one position around twenty hours per day, day after day while your scalp perspires. I don't know about you, but the back of my head produced a bird's nest that could only be extracted a few strands at a time.

Here's a solution: braid it or hold it off your neck in plastic or rubber bands (metal clips might not be allowed in surgery).

But don't chop it off. Reclaiming your look is part of recovery, so keep your beautiful hair. You *will* be well enough to take care of it again.

Sex

My eighty-year-old aunt, who works as a sex therapist for severely disabled adults, reminds me that any place on the body that can feel, can feel sexual. Her paralyzed patient, whose only sensation is above his neck, has sensual experiences with his ears and his scalp. No, back surgery survivors are not consigned to the sexiness of hair conditioners, but in the early months out of the hospital I doubt your sex life will be what it once was.

Nurses from the spine unit advise that couples may resume sex as soon as three weeks after surgery using the "missionary position," flat on your back or lying side by side. I can't speak for men. But, women, let's talk: You're not going to want this. Unless pain is a turn-on, you won't feel interested when your back hurts, you feel queasy, your abdomen is bloated, and the hospital smell has lingered, dissipating only gradually through your pores. You can't bend, twist, lean, or carry any weight, and you might have trouble lifting your legs and moving them.

But take heart — life will improve. Women who had this operation years ago tell me they can now do just about anything they want. And remember my aunt. Nobody operated on your head!

Exercise: Preparation

I prepared for surgery the way a runner might train for a marathon. Okay, in truth, it was more like the way a non-runner would exercise enough to stay in the pack, glad to make it past the finish line at all. In retrospect, I wish I'd done more.

My goals were shaped by what I'd heard from former spine patients: one lost 20 pounds, mostly muscle, while he was in the hospital; several said they couldn't lift their legs to step over the ledge into the shower; many told me they shuffled along with tiny steps at first; and everyone felt exhausted.

My plan was: Pilates to target "core" muscles, mostly the abdominals to help lift my legs and walk. A while back I'd attended Mat Pilates classes at the gym, but not until I'd found a professional Pilates studio with trained instructors and a full range of equipment did I understand it. For six months at Retrofit Pilates in Santa Monica, California, I worked with Gaida, a teacher who was a ballerina, originally from Latvia. She focused on perfect positioning during specific movements that seemed to stretch my spine by using muscles to support it in alignment. She also worked on my mid-back, which had been rigid when I'd begun. Whatever flexibility I could achieve might make the surgery easier, we reasoned, when it was time for the doctor to straighten my spine.

I can hear her admonishing, "Grow taller, taller, taller — yes!" After half a century of walking, now I was learning to walk. When I walked down the street I became aware of my abdominals moving up, and holding the crown of my head to the sky like, well, a ballet dancer.

A few weeks before surgery, the owner of Retrofit was so enthusiastic she urged me to have new X-rays to see if they'd actually improved my spine. No, of course they hadn't. Neither

Pilates nor any other exercise can fix a 68-degree curve, but the concentrated training two days a week for six months had improved my strength and may have warded off back pain before the operation. And I learned how my body works in ways no one else had shown me.

For years I'd practiced yoga with a wonderfully obsessed yoga master who taught a class of five people. Each of them would have been ordinary except that they'd shown up for intense 90-minute sessions for so many years they were standing on their heads and gliding from "downward dog" to an array of poses suitable for Gumby or other rubber beings. For a while, I'd kept up with the others, but in the years before surgery as my spine declined by a degree each year, I found my pelvis was bumping into my rib cage, and one by one, I had to sit out the poses. Finally, I quit.

I downgraded to yoga at the gym, where every inch of floor was claimed by someone's towel. Here, I figured I'd do what I could, and hide the rest of the time. Personally, I don't recommend that kind of mass yoga. You could injure yourself if you're not holding a pose properly, and no one would notice. Anyway, I was becoming too physically limited, even for this group.

I wish I'd continued the hip-opening moves, though. After surgery, when I could no longer bend, being able to move my hip to the side and elevate my foot to the opposite thigh (as in the lotus position) would be essential to maintaining a relationship with my feet. I should mention, though, that my pelvis is not fused, so my hips can move. If you're fused down to your pelvis, this probably won't be an option.

Besides Pilates twice a week, I intended to go to the gym three other days. I said "intended." Sometimes I got there twice; on busy weeks, only once. I pushed myself on the treadmill, hoping I'd release endorphins, though I often didn't succeed. When I didn't get to the gym I walked a mile or so each day. All that's really not much, but I was increasing my stamina at least a little.

I was afraid of upper body weight-training because I couldn't risk compressing my spine, but if I could have afforded it, I would have hired a personal trainer at the gym. If your back is degenerating, as mine was, the risk of worsening the pressure on discs, or that your spine might actually give way altogether, is real. A professional might have provided the security to grow stronger safely.

Working by myself on the treadmill, bikes, and various leg-lift machines built quads (thigh muscles) that I needed more than I'd anticipated. Now, if I'm on a soft low chair and I can't reach anything to pull myself up, or a hard surface from which to push off, my only resource has been these tough thighs (which women often lament as "too big"). Placing my hands on my upper legs, I can stand using the thigh muscles alone. If I couldn't, I'd still be sitting there, waiting to be rescued.

Similarly, deep knee bends allow you to pick up stuff from the floor, especially if you don't have your "grabber." Remember, you can't lean over, so your only means of reaching earth and standing again is by working those thighs.

In hindsight, I wish I'd developed other muscles too. Lying in bed for weeks, my hamstrings (in back of my legs) began to shorten. When hamstrings are tight, it's difficult to straighten your legs. And the stress of taking steps on legs that won't lift or reach forward might send pain up into your lower back. The remedy is stretching, and if I'd known then what I know now, I would have lengthened those rubber bands plenty.

I also wish I'd improved my arms. It didn't seem relevant before surgery, but when I was stuck in bed and my back and abs were too damaged to move me, the only way to turn or roll or lift up from the bed was to push with my arms. I'm told that men have greater upper body strength, so this might be easy for them. But if your shoulders aren't flexible and your arms can't bear your weight (as in push-ups), you're stuck flat in that bed like a flounder.

But please don't beat yourself up for having only 24 hours in a day, or having to go to work. Whatever you can do, do it, and that will help.

Exercise: Recovery

"What am I supposed to do about rehab?" I asked Dr. Pashman, four months after surgery.

"What are you doing?" he responded.

"Walking a lot, Pilates twice a week and I guess I'll start back at the gym."

"Then that's your rehab," he said.

So I'm sorry I can't share my experience with professional rehabilitation. I do know that my hospital, like many others, offers a swimming pool and specialists who work one-on-one with patients; and I hear that people benefit, especially those who have difficulty walking. However, several former patients told me they designed their own programs, especially those who were active before surgery. Getting back your full function — and more — is an individual journey. The question isn't where or by which method, but how strong do you care enough to become?

One former patient told me he was advised to use a Nordic Trak-type treadmill. So he bought an expensive one and placed it grandly in front of his TV. I asked if that worked for him.

"I'm sure it would," he said, "but I'd have to use the thing. I don't like doing exercise."

So he was still creeping around a year later. Really, this phase is up to you, but I can offer the physical issues I targeted in case you have these too: blown abs, tight legs, shallow breathing, lousy stamina and weak muscle tone — each of which seems to compound the others.

Abs: When a surgeon accesses the spine from the front, he has to separate the abdominal muscles. I'm told the muscles aren't cut through, but he slices along the natural divisions so they can be moved aside. After surgery, I sported a huge tummy bulge and didn't know if that was swelling, or weird muscles, or scar tissue.

A scar would have been the worst because I'd have to live with a tire circling my front forever. If the cause was post-op swelling, I reasoned, the area would deflate in the first month or so. And yes, the swelling did subside, though that took three months.

In its wake was still a rubbery ridge across my front below my navel — the terrain of the cut that led to my departed rib. So I was relieved to learn the culprits are muscles. Okay, I thought, if they're alive, they can be molded.

But as for normal abs exercises, especially crunches, sit-ups, and those impossible twists where you touch your elbow to your opposite knee — fuhgeddaboutit. If you've had a surgery like mine, you can't do those, and even if you somehow could, you shouldn't. That kind of violent twisting could wrench the screws from your bones and break the steel rods.

Instead, Gaida, my Pilates teacher, has me using my own force while standing or lying flat. The effort isn't only to pull in; it's also aimed upwards, more of a rolling motion. Besides that, I work flat on my back to protect my spine while I do various leg lifts that impact the "core" muscles. Everywhere I walk, I hear Gaida's voice reminding me to work my gut.

Tight legs: Lying and sitting around for months did in my hamstrings and calves. At first I could barely straighten my legs to walk and I sure couldn't lift them. This is simply about stretching little by little, and as long as you take it slowly and take care to keep your back straight, you can easily find leg stretches. What matters is not so much the regimen you choose but how well it releases you to reach a longer stride that fights that post-op shuffle. People in professional rehab, or who have a pool, have told me that walking through waist-deep water was helpful too.

Breathing: I came home with shallow breaths and a rattle in my left lung that had collapsed in surgery. Despite the admonitions of nurses to inhale into a little plastic device to make tiny balls lift, I didn't improve much in the first month. Without good aeration, my energy wasn't likely to increase, not to mention that I was risking pneumonia. But what to do? I know one woman who took up singing lessons. She said singing not only deepened her breathing but made her feel like she was having fun instead of being rehabilitated. I confess, though, I didn't do much about breathing (except to keep doing it), and after four months I was pretty much okay anyway.

As for overall stamina and tone, my doctor recommended basic cardio: walking and using a treadmill. He warned me against a regular bike, concerned the forward lean would stress my spine, but he said a recumbent bike with a back support would be okay.

More important than choosing this or that machine, I suggest you decide on your overall intention. For me, this process wasn't only about recovering from surgery; it was about being a healthy person engaging a challenging world. From that idea, once you determine to be strong, you'll find many ways.

A Good Attitude

When you're planning major surgery everyone and their uncle advises you to "be positive" and "have a good attitude." My friends insist the reason I recovered so well was that my attitude was good. I don't even know what the heck that means.

The platitude elicits a creepy image of a round yellow happy face with lame-brained dot eyes and a lipless smile pasted over someone in pain; in other words, a phony. It also conjures people who deny their own ability to take charge of their situation by asserting "I'll be fine" while affecting a beatific smile, their glazed-over eyes looking down on those who don't believe that faith is sufficient so they don't have to do anything. I'm sorry, in my opinion, that won't get you through this surgery.

What you need is truth and a strong dose of your own power. Truth, not artificial sweeteners, because only when you know what's actually going on can you own this experience enough to manage it. And you need guts. It takes courage to plan this surgery and thoroughly prepare for any eventuality, including disabling pain or even death; courage to force yourself to move your body immediately afterwards; courage to reclaim your life in a changed body. It takes both physical and mental strength to persevere by holding to a clear vision of what you want to do.

Not to be grandiose, but I'd even advise you to verbalize what you're living for. I recommend being specific. Instead of a facile answer like "for my family," try to define distinct, tangible desires and goals, which may involve asking questions about what you really want. Sure, it's a biggie; it's like asking who you truly are.

I went out and gathered particular art supplies down to a new rich golden yellow paint called "light orange," a name that doesn't capture what it promised me. I bought materials in various sizes, in case I might have to start small, and a whole new bottle of glossy acrylic painting medium. My daughter, the singer, had scheduled shows after my surgery and those dates became targets for me to attend. John and I wanted to improve our cracked-cement patio with tiles, and I picked out the style before I went to the hospital, though the renovation would be months away. And I began writing this book.

Your plans for joy after you recover might surprise you — they're not only about being safely home and getting back to work; maybe they're what you've always wanted. I hope you make those plans. It helps to focus on them when you're feeling bad.

As for attitude, I prefer the image of gripping the metal railing on the side of the hospital bed with all my might to be able to roll off a bedpan, how much arm strength that took, and how much will to persevere was required when the pain cut through me like a blade. Yes, I'd rather offer that crude example as a guide rather than an image of someone lying helpless in bed pleading to the darkness to make her better some day.

Listen, nobody gets out of life alive. But you can win this round. First, don't be shy about being your own advocate. Your questions aren't stupid and anyone who acts annoyed is a jerk. Get the answers you need (though a nurse might help as well as your doctor, and probably has more time). Complain if something's wrong, even if you discover it's a normal phase of healing and you simply have to go through it. That happened to me when I felt more pain at seven weeks than I'd had three weeks after surgery.

And keep moving. My brother, the doctor, once commented that a leading cause of death is sitting down. He wasn't entirely joking: At the time we were talking about osteoporosis and how a hip fracture may lead to a wheelchair where the immobility cascades into other problems that can hasten death. Of course, you're not running marathons right after surgery. In fact, you must respect the healing process; let it take its natural course. But over time, if you give up, your body will give up on you.

So what's a good attitude? For me, it meant getting in shape in the months before surgery with an exercise program. It meant being aware of the strange chemicals that would invade my body during the surgeries, and that I'd need to eat in a way that made me as resilient as possible on entering, and to cleanse my system after I was home. It involved trying to walk soon after surgery, no matter how difficult that was. Later, I walked further and further with longer steps each day, and finally I went back to Pilates and a cardio program.

To me, all that is an affirmation that energy will continue to move within you. But it won't move by itself, so get out of bed and off that chair and go for it. That's the great "yes" to your future. That's the good attitude I wish for you.

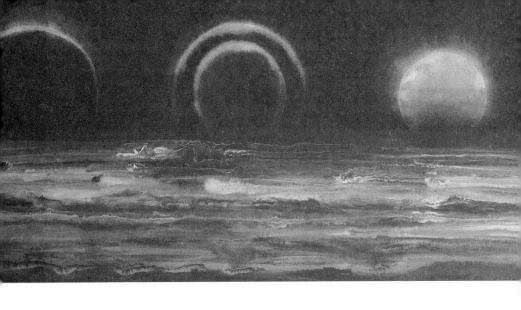

Appendix II

Interviews with
Dr. Robert Pashman, M.D.

Director, Scoliosis and Spinal Deformity
Institute for Spinal Disorders,
Cedars-Sinai Medical Center

I INTERVIEWED MY DOCTOR TWICE. The first time was soon after the surgery in 2005 when I visited him in his office, following my final visit as a patient. It felt odd to see him in his office rather than an exam room, and to talk as one professional to another — he, not in a lab coat and me, not in a hospital gown or even a brace. He was solicitous that I sit in a comfortable chair — the operation had been only months before — but I waved him off and headed for the most daunting lounge chair in the room — tough; not wanting to be vulnerable anymore.

I asked the kinds of journalistic questions that might frame any research subject: *Why are you in this work? What is the history? What projects are you focusing on? Where is your field going?* For someone who had taken me through such a personal journey, it was perhaps a distancing effort, a way to have a handle on it all, to place him as my equal. Of course, to the doctor, it was an aspect of patient education or outreach, without the coloration of fear or transformation, without a hint of what it had meant to me.

That first interview from 2005 follows. Just the facts, solid information, like dry land after a storm.

PD: Why did you choose this field? What does it mean to you?

PASHMAN: Spine orthopedic surgery is fascinating in the sense that it's like carpentry. It's gratifying because bones heal. It's rewarding because you can make a very positive impact, but it's my impression that not all patients are created equal. Many patients have psychological problems going into the surgery and their expectations are influenced by that. If you have scoliosis your whole life, you're shaped psychologically as well as physically.

Number one is the cosmetic aspect, especially for girls who think they're deformed. They may feel that the way they look is the explanation for why they don't get certain jobs, why they have painful backs, why they have a difficult time with friends, and other problems. If you're a sixteen-year-old who has to wear a brace, you can imagine the psychosocial impact — you'd have issues of confinement and isolation. Major studies have documented a difference in marital rates between patients who have scoliosis and who don't have scoliosis. There have also been studies that try to show whether or not patients with scoliosis have a higher propensity to have back pain as they get older.

Having said that, I have to say that in 2005, and probably for the last ten years, most patients don't get to be adults with big curves because most of those kids are identified and then have surgery as kids. Now, adult scoliosis is not as common as adolescent scoliosis. For that same reason, adult scoliosis is more common in non-urban areas than urban areas because the degree of medical sophistication is higher here.

My best experience is with patients who come into surgery mentally prepared, in good physical condition, willing to do what they have to do, and who understand that if in fact they don't do something to treat their scoliosis they're going to get worse over time, and then it can be very hard to deal with.

Of course, it's always gratifying to operate on children because, unlike adults, their spines are very flexible and you can place them anywhere you want. Think about a thirteen or fourteen year old adolescent girl who has a deformity like an elevated shoulder blade or a hump in her back, or something like that, and you give her the cosmetic benefit of stopping the progression.

PD: What are some problems you've had?

PASHMAN: There are limitations to what we can do. In the case of a woman who, after the change of life has osteoporosis, there's only so much you can do in terms of screws and rods being able to manipulate the spine. The screws might not hold, so you have to know your limitations. Not only is the surgery more difficult, but the complications of heart rate and other health problems also goes up when you deal with older patients, just because they're older.

Fortunately, I've never paralyzed a patient, which would be a devastating complication. That's because we're very careful. We monitor nerves, and in the old days we used to wake patients up in the middle of the operation to move their feet. We're very careful about how we do things, so that has not happened. I've never had a death.

The problems I've had, which are pretty common, are that the patient doesn't heal, and then I have to take them back and put them on something so they will heal. The signs of not healing can be that the curve gets worse over time, even after the rods. Or a rod breaks. Or the patient has pain which is not really explained by anything else.

Each patient signs a consent form that says there may be complications of surgery, and what the percentages are. All the spine surgeons who belong to the Scoliosis Research Society are supposed to submit their complications on a periodic basis. That data is taken worldwide and boiled down to a statistical understanding of what the complication rate is for all the surgeries. It turns out that the complication rate for neurological problems (pinched nerves or spinal cord injuries) is probably less than half a percent; infections 1%; mortality is probably less than .3%. Of course it depends on how old the patient is and the severity of their problems.

PD: What got you into this? Can you tell me something about the history of this operation?

PASHMAN: I first became interested during one of my rotations in medical school. I met a guy who was doing pediatric orthopedics. Just like many things in life, it can all be boiled down to one mentor, one person who makes such a great impact on your life that it molds you. That's who this guy was for me. He did spine surgery on kids and I decided very early on that I wanted to do spine surgery, maybe my second or third year.

I knew I had to do a fellowship because spine surgery is almost its own discipline. I went to a program at the University of Minnesota, which was the most famous scoliosis place on the planet from 1955 to maybe 1990. All of scoliosis or deformity surgery really had its roots in about five men. Everybody who does this type of surgery is descended from those five guys — it's like six degrees of separation.

One of those guys who started this deformity program was the pinnacle. His name is John Moe. Thousands of people are descended from him. So for two years I studied in Minnesota, and then I followed one of John Moe's greatest students to San Francisco and did my clinical work at the University of California, San Francisco.

When I came to Los Angeles in 1992, there were no spine surgeons. Nobody was doing this. Of course, since that time, spine surgery has grown and has broken down into a lot of components: back pain, neck pain, sciatica, and what I do. The lion's share of my practice is major deformity, including scoliosis and kyphosis, which is like humpback.

As there became more doctors in the community who did spine surgery, my practice became super-specialized. Not too many people like doing this because it's very complicated. It's big surgery. Usually I have to rely on other doctors to work with me during surgery and for other specialties. There's an art to operating on scoliosis so the patient is perfectly balanced. That requires three-dimensional visualization and a lot of experience. We train surgeons right here — we call them fellows. These are guys who've already finished their residency and want a year of the spine training.

Now I have patients who fly here from all over the place ... Boston ... China. They think I know what I'm doing. Cedars-Sinai is a good hospital and Los Angeles is a mecca of medicine. So if patients have a complicated surgery like scoliosis they may well look outside their own areas. In fairness, many people have been trained since I began, and they go to local communities. The difference is that, in my career, I've done probably close to 1200 major deformity cases. That comes out to about a hundred each year.

PD: And you do research also....

PASHMAN: Yes, I do basic science research on the cause of scoliosis. I got a grant from a foundation, and so I go every year and sit on a panel of six researchers from around the world to talk about the causation of scoliosis. Believe it or not, we know how to treat it, but we don't know what causes it. Some of the theories are that it's genetic, and we know that because it goes from mother to daughter, for example. There are abnormalities in the inner ear and balance. There are abnormalities in certain types of genes.

My research has to do with the cerebrospinal fluid flow in patients with scoliosis. We're currently doing that research here. In other words, the flow of the fluid around the spinal cord is different in curved spines. We now know it would affect brain function, but the issue is whether or not that flow is different because of the scoliosis or if it actually makes the scoliosis worse. Theoretically, if this flow made the scoliosis worse, potentially we can do something to alter the flow, which might stop the scoliosis — like have the patient blow up a balloon, or subject the patient to some sort of magnetic field, or something like that.

There have also been studies about muscle strength on one side of the curve as opposed to the center, but we really don't know what causes it.

PD: Looking towards the future, what's the prognosis for treating people with spine deformities?

PASHMAN: The ultimate future is to prevent it. That's not happening so soon because we don't know what causes it. In scoliosis surgery the advances are basically in the types of instrumentation that we use. One very interesting thing that is happening, at least in children, is that we might be able to manipulate the growth on one side of the spine so we stop growth on one side while the other side catches up, which could stop the curve, and that might be done by minimally invasive means.

Things like artificial discs, for example, will probably never be relevant to scoliosis because the progression of the curvature is not amenable. The technology that is applicable to low back pain such as gene therapy, growing discs in the laboratory, making mechanical discs, and all the other things that we do for low back pain in general are probably not applicable to scoliosis and deformity surgery. It doesn't make sense to wait for science to advance for scoliosis because in five or ten years the curve will get worse, and it just becomes harder to fix. There is a time element that supersedes the technology.

PD: From your point of view, what makes a good patient, or a difficult patient?

PASHMAN: Well, you understood that from the first time you saw your X-ray and we discussed your options. You were the best kind of patient because you weren't taking pain medications going into the surgery, so your endorphin levels, which are the natural painkillers in the body, were maximized. Not only that, but you were in good physical health. And from a psychological standpoint you seemed to be on a very even keel, without an overtly depressive side. You did your homework. You felt comfortable with your surgeon. And you had a very good support system. All of those things together, plus realistic expectations about what you'd be going through, and knowing why you were doing this, added up to the best possible kind of patient to operate on.

The worst patient would be exactly the opposite. I have had some patients who were not so much big deformity patients, but who wanted cosmetic changes or who expected me to cure their back pain after they'd been on tremendous amounts of pain medication for many years. My feeling is that they would still be on pain medicine after I operated so what's the point? To me, one goal of the surgery is a narcotic-free life. I don't think there's anything wrong with taking pain medicine if it's under a doctor's prescription, if that's what you need. But if I can turn a patient who depends on narcotics into a patient who doesn't take drugs, and they feel better, that's what I would do.

A lot of the surgery we do is not only for pain or deformity but also for function. In other words, if the patient is crippled by their pain and we can make them more productive, able to do things they want, such as travel or whatever they hope to do, then that is a good outcome. A lot of patients are debilitated by their pain, so I operate on them — if I can get them so that they can do more things, then that's a good outcome.

To go out walking is the ultimate. For me, if I can return that function to somebody, that's the greatest success.

MY SECOND INTERVIEW WITH DR. PASHMAN was five years later in August 2010. He was busy and did me the favor of fitting me in with a phone call between patients, so my final contact was taping a disembodied voice coming out of a tiny grid on the telephone speaker. I merely intended to update the information for readers of this book. I wanted to know if leaps had occurred in spine operations. I was curious to hear if his ideas had changed, or if there were stories of other patients. But the conversation brought me back into the world of the surgery years after I was over it. The technicalities, procedures, considerations of timing and the measurement of results — perfect, of course, for necessary information, but infinitely far from where I am now.

PD: Since the last time I spoke with you, are there innovations or techniques you've discovered? Are there procedures you do differently from what you did five years ago?

PASHMAN: We basically do almost exactly the same thing. The techniques are approximately the same but we have some innovations in terms of how we do those things. In the last year and a half we've been using a device called the "O-Arm." It's an intra-operative CT-scan. We take the information from the CT-scanner and feed it into a computer that tells us where to put the screws. You have screws. We still use screws. We use the same strategy and we would do the same operation on you, except, instead of using X-rays to help us put the screws in, we now have a computer put them in for us.

PD: Besides that technical change, have you noticed any difference in the conversations you have with patients or their expectations?

PASHMAN: We manage expectations now through advances on my website [*www.espine.com*]. It has everything patients need to know pre- and post-operatively so we communicate a little differently. We offer these educational materials through my website where patients get themselves up to speed. Expectation management is the key to success. The way we communicate is by the website which has graphics and calendars. But the indications, the goals, the strategy, the actual operation — everything we do is basically the same as when you had your operation.

PD: Are as many people having spine surgery now?

PASHMAN: We find that people who have severe scoliosis like yourself now know and can find people who specialize and do it all the time. So, once they have that level of comfort that there are people in their city who do this kind of operation all the time, they're much more amenable to doing it from a confidence level. Our practice, which is adult and adolescent idiopathic scoliosis, has seen no change in the people who are seeking out this type of operation and I think that's a trend across the country.

PD: Are there future trends or experiences you've had in the last five years readers might like to know about?

PASHMAN: Who knows if society is going to be tolerant of doing these expensive operations? That's the first consideration. Private insurers may scrutinize these operations from cost considerations. Who knows what's going to happen in that respect. People who have adult scoliosis need to be pro-active in thinking about whether they're going to be able to have these reconstructions, and the freedom they're going to have from them, in terms of insurance coverage.

The second consideration is that all these spine operations would in the best possible world be done in ways that are easier on patients. There are lasers and minimally invasive treatments. The problem with adult scoliosis — big curves like you had — we're talking about an architectural, engineering problem. If you have a building that's falling over you can't put chewing gum on it.

A lot of the things that need to be done when you have big curves require a certain quantity of force applied to the spine. Any trend that has to do with artificial discs — motion preservation, or is minimally invasive — putting in things by robot and so forth — is not going to be used for adult scoliosis like you had because so much force has to be applied to get these things corrected and balanced. Although the trends in medicine are through smaller incisions, the trend in adult scoliosis has lagged behind that because we're dealing with a different kind of situation.

PD: Is there a difference in children's scoliosis?

PASHMAN: This is my philosophy about children's scoliosis — I've had this conversation with my colleagues who do pediatric orthopedics: If you have a 13-year-old who has a large curve, and a 25-year-old who has a large curve, and a 35-year-old who has a large curve, I would correct the 13-year-old, the 25-year-old and the 35-year-old the same way. With the modern techniques, I can get the same corrections at 13, 25 and 35. The question is: why is it important to tell parents that their kids have to have surgery at 13? At least they can have the option of the surgery when they're a freshman in high school, a junior, a senior, between high school and college years, or after college, or even when they're into their career. I think that's the trend.

The other side of the argument I've heard from the pediatric surgeons is that the kids are easier because the spine is so flexible, and kids have family support. But I'm predicting that options for patients will be much larger in the future because of timing, because the techniques have advanced so far that we're as good at correcting scoliosis at all age levels, given the same size curve.

PD: What about much older adults? Is that prognosis still good?

PASHMAN: It is good, but it has to be balanced. Even though the techniques are safer, when a patient is older they have to accept the chance of higher risk in the late 50s, 60s and 70s. The complication rates go up as patients get older. Also, the biology of bone softening and cardiovascular effects change as people get older. So, patients have to talk to their doctor. They have to get the pros and cons of surgery at each age. If they want to wait, that's their prerogative, but there might be higher risk.

PD: If someone was contemplating back surgery and they're not in Los Angeles, and they're frightened, and having back pain, and they have severe scoliosis, what should they do?

PASHMAN: They should realize that back pain is different from scoliosis. Everybody has low back pain. If you have low back pain you can have it treated on a local level. Low back pain rarely needs surgery. But once you have scoliosis, spinal deformity, you have to realize these are very complicated operations. The most important thing is to find people who have the most experience to do these operations, wherever they are geographically. The reason we're so successful is that we have teams. We have the same anesthesiologist, for example, everybody doing the same techniques over and over. You want to go to a place with a high volume, where an experienced team does surgery, and that may not be in someone's hometown. They're going to have to seek out a major center. Every metropolitan area has a hospital where somebody does high volume scoliosis surgery.

PD: Is there a final word of wisdom you'd like to share?

PASHMAN: From the standpoint of safety and technology, this type of treatment — the surgical treatment for scoliosis — is getting better and better. It's getting safer and being applied to patients on a much wider age basis. So the real issue is that there's hope. The hope is that you don't have to be hunched over and you don't have to have scoliosis to the point that you're totally dysfunctional. There are safe, effective treatments for these things, and that in itself inspires people.

Resources

≈

IF YOU SEARCH THE INTERNET for Spine Surgery, Back Surgery, Spine Fusion, Scoliosis or Spinal Deformity or any combination, you will find page after page of listings — hundreds of websites on the subject. Some are support organizations, some are physician networks, some are individual doctors and hospitals who do these operations. And some are — well — I really don't think your back problems were caused by space aliens!

If you are looking for experienced doctors or medical centers anywhere in the world, or want to learn more before embarking on this operation, my doctor recommends starting with these four reliable sources:

Scoliosis Research Society: *www.SRS.org*
American Society of Orthopedic Surgeons: *www.AAOS.org*
The Scoliosis Foundation: *www.TheScoliosisFoundation.org*
Dr. Pashman's website: *www.espine.com*
Spine-Health: *www.spine-health.com*

Image Credits

≈

Paintings by Pam Douglas:

Pg. 1: *Tracks*, 2008, 20" × 40", acrylic on raw linen

Pg. 9: *The Road Ahead*, 2008, 20" × 40", acrylic on raw linen

Pg. 45: *The Kite Flyer*, 2009, 50" × 16", mixed media on raw linen

Pg. 93: *Messages*, 2007, 20" × 20", acrylic on raw linen

Pg. 145: *The Horizon Line*, 2009, 40" × 20", acrylic on raw linen

Pg. 151: *Life Lines* (diptych), 2009, 32" × 30", mixed media on raw linen

Pg. 167: *I Shall Return with the Tide*, 2008, 20" × 40", acrylic on raw linen

About Pamela Douglas

≈

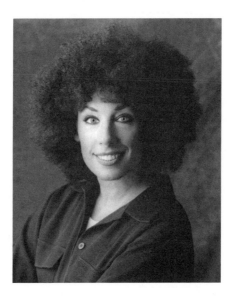

PAMELA DOUGLAS is an award-winning writer with numerous credits in television drama. The Second Edition of her book, *Writing the TV Drama Series* (Michael Wiese Productions 2007), has been translated into many languages and, with a third edition due out in 2011, is considered the premiere book on the subject.

Pamela has been honored with the Humanitas Prize for *Between Mother and Daughter* (CBS), an original drama which also won a nomination for a Writers Guild Award. Multiple Emmy nominations and awards, and awards from American Women in Radio and Television, went to other dramas she has written.

Pamela has been a member of the Board of Directors of the Writers Guild of America (West), and is a tenured professor in the screenwriting division at the School of Cinematic Arts of the University of Southern California.

She is also a painter and has exhibited widely, including at the Los Angeles County Museum of Art (Sales & Rental Gallery). Her art is represented by TAG Gallery at the prestigious Bergamot Station Art Center in Santa Monica, CA.

Contact Pamela Douglas at
www.PamDouglasBooks.com,
www.PamDouglasArt.com, and *pamdouglaswords@aol.com.*

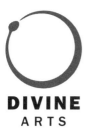

DIVINE
A R T S

DIVINE ARTS sprang to life fully formed as an intention to bring spiritual practice into daily living. Human beings are far more than the one-dimensional creatures perceived by most of humanity and held static in consensus reality. There is a deep and vast body of knowledge — both ancient and emerging — that informs and gives us the understanding, through direct experience, that we are magnificent creatures occupying many dimensions with untold powers and connectedness to all that is. Divine Arts books and films explore these realms, powers and teachings through inspiring, informative and empowering works by pioneers, artists and great teachers from all the wisdom traditions.

We invite your participation and look forward to learning how we may better serve you.

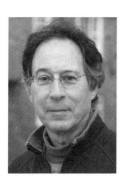

Onward and upward,

Michael Wiese
Publisher/Filmmaker

DivineArtsMedia.com